Praise for *Speaking in Tongues*

In her autobiography Speaking in Tongues, *renowned scholar Fedwa Malti-Douglas displays a poet's eye for evocative imagery, summoning up the Lebanon of her childhood and a novelist's mastery of compelling storytelling. This radiant, revelatory book demonstrates how narrative nonfiction can accommodate the coincidences and astonishing plot twists of the nineteenth-century novel (her beloved Dickens comes to mind) simply because it's required to stick to the facts and faithfully report whatever happens, however surprising those reversals of fortune and reappearances of characters may be. Her book's title refers most obviously to her command of several languages, but it's still remarkable that the English in which she composes her life story is her third language, after Arabic and French, and that she was forced to learn it upon her arrival in America at the age of thirteen. This self-portrait is courageous in its frankness about the pain from both her inherited Charcot-Marie-Tooth disease, a form of muscular dystrophy, and her Post-Traumatic Stress Disorder. Despite all sorts of suffering, most of it following the "erupting volcano" of her father's death, Fedwa Malti-Douglas exults in the felicities of her richly complicated life.*

John Drury
Author of *Sea Level Rising*

Speaking in Tongues *is a vibrant autobiography. Cinematic and luscious, it is also heartbreaking as we travel with our true-life narrator from innocence to experience. Fedwa Malti-Douglas's shocking and well-wrought narrative reads like a combination of Proust's* In Search of Lost Time *and Charlotte Bronte's* Jane Eyre. *She evokes her childhood in Deir el-Amar, the "Abode of the Moon," stunningly, the cough drops she knew as a child (those French pastilles) bringing time back in a burst of sweetness. When her father dies, leaving his money and huge estate to his brother in America, the downward movement of her changing circumstances is inexorable. The contrast is fairy-tale stark, her uncle serving as evil stepfather. Her escape is made possible by a love of books and hard work in college. In graduate school, Fedwa discovers that she has inherited not only her father's brilliance but a rare type of muscular dystrophy, the reason why her aunt in Lebanon had legs like "upside-down champagne bottles." This wise and honest book leaves us not with some romanticized framing of the past but the knowledge that "the past is an essential part of the future, albeit a past that must be tamed."*

LaWanda Walters
Author of *Light Is the Odalisque*

Fedwa Malti-Douglas's Speaking in Tongues *is a deeply moving and arresting account of her painful but heroic journey from a Christian childhood in a Lebanese village (where her father was a physician and her mother had deserted the family) to teen-age life in Ithaca, New York, where her Cornell professor uncle regularly beat both her and her brother, to a brilliant university career in Middle Eastern Studies. This was made difficult by the onset of an hereditary muscular dystrophy that Fedwa Malti and her historian husband Allen Douglas have battled with extraordinary bravery. As one reads this riveting narrative, one wonders how the author managed, despite all hardships, and retain her sense of humor and optimism and her love of nature and art. Both fierce and funny, Fedwa is a role model for us all!*

Marjorie Perloff
Author of *The Vienna Paradox*
Sadie D. Patek Professor Emerita of Humanities, Stanford University
Presidential Fellow, Chapman University

In Speaking in Tongues, *Fedwa Malti-Douglas has given us a memoir of unpitying clarity. The pasts she explores are intellectual, physical, and emotional; her own and her extended family's; local and trans-cultural. In tight, economical prose, she lingers only on the most telling details of habit and custom, diet and ritual, attraction and estrangement. The very act of writing brings the recollection into being, its emotional intensity coming into focus on one central narrative: that of a family lost and regained.*

Gregory Woods
Nottingham Trent University
Author of *An Ordinary Dog* and *A History of Gay Literature*

So many memoirs of the past fifteen or so years have struck me cold—fulfilling little more than a kind of intellectual secretion, full of self-pity and self-justification as if the self were the holy grail of existence. Fedwa Malti-Douglas's Speaking in Tongues *is beautifully self-deprecating, honest—even confiding—without the slightest hint of complaint or self-glorification. I wish I could "speak in tongues," because I would be doing just that for this intelligent, thoughtful journey through a uniquely American life. Yes, I said that. And how desperately we need citizens like this brave scholar and poet.*

Richard Bausch
Professor in the Writing Program
at Chapman University in Orange, California
Author of *Peace*
and *Before, During, After*

"Speaking in tongues is one gift; understanding the words is another..." says Malti-Douglas's mother of her unusual talent. But the author's own quest to understand the words that articulate her origin story is yet another type of gift, one bestowed upon her readers.

From a fairytale-like childhood set in her physician father's lemon tree–lined Lebanese estate, to her forced immigration—at 13 years of age—to a battering uncle's home in Miami, Florida, Malti-Douglas bravely navigates the roiling waters of her personal journey.

Loving her adopted country as only an immigrant who appreciates all it has to offer can, *the missing puzzle pieces of the author's past nevertheless continue to obsess her. She wills her increasingly uncooperative—and finally wheelchair-bound body—to press from coast to coast, continent to continent, fueled by a desire to satisfy her ravenous appetite to reconnect with the heritage from which she'd been prematurely torn.*

When she finally succeeds in sitting down to break bread with her long-lost relatives, it's in dazzling style—here was akhtaboot, kofta, tamriyya, *and* baked kibbee in enormous pans cut into lovely diamonds—*not unlike like the dazzling facets of Malti-Douglas's prose. If it all sounds immensely intoxicating, it's because it is.*

Lissa Kiernan
Author of *Two Faint Lines in the Violet*
and *Glass Needles & Goose Quills*

In Speaking in Tongues *celebrated scholar Fedwa Malti-Douglas renders the past visible, almost palpable, by the sheer power of love. This remarkable autobiography is a chronicle of one of our living intellectual heroines who struggled with entrenched thoughts that chained the bodies and minds of women across various continents and oceans, who wrestled with ghosts that aimed to defeat her will and an illness that challenged her remarkable spirit. It is a search of times past that preserves the future of valor and dignity.*

Khaled Mattawa
Author of *Tocqueville* and *Amorisco*
Professor of English Language and Literature, University of Michigan

Almost Proustian in her patience, Fedwa Malti-Douglas offers up a life story that is as intellectually rigorous as it is sensuous. There are so many kinds of invisibility, and here, Dr. Malti-Douglas gives shape to so many. Her writing— smart, poetic and often revelatory—is blessed with what Walter Benjamin calls the "optical unconscious," revealing what lurks in putative plain sight, what we choose not to see. Modeling a life fully lived despite astonishing hardships astonishingly born, she bears us from Lebanon to the US to Mexico and back. Speaking in Tongues *carries us on a journey that crosses landscapes of sadness, of happiness, of pain and peace, of alienation and acceptance, toward a healing enlargement of the soul. We are enlightened voyagers.*

Jeffrey Levine
Poet and author of *Rumor of Cortez*
Editor, Tupelo Press

Speaking in Tongues

Speaking in Tongues

Fedwa Malti-Douglas

The American Philosophical
Society Press

Philadelphia • 2017

TRANSACTIONS OF THE
AMERICAN PHILOSOPHICAL SOCIETY
HELD AT PHILADELPHIA
FOR PROMOTING USEFUL KNOWLEDGE
VOLUME 106, PART 4

ISBN 978-1-60618-064-8

US ISSN 978-1-60618-066-2

Library of Congress Cataloging-in Publication Data

Names: Malti-Douglas, Fedwa, author.
Title: Speaking in tongues / Fedwa Malti-Douglas.
Description: Philadelphia : American Philosophical Society, 2017. | Series:
  Transactions of the American Philosophical Society, ISSN 0065-9746 ;
  volume 105, part 1
Identifiers: LCCN 2017000738| ISBN 9781606180648 (paperback) | ISBN
  9781606180662 (ebook)
Subjects: LCSH: Malti-Douglas, Fedwa. | Women scholars–United
  States–Biography. | Scholars–United States–Biography. | Middle
  East–Study and teaching (Higher)–United States. | Indiana University,
  Bloomington–Faculty–Biography. | Lebanese Americans–Biography. |
  Christians–Lebanon–Biography. | Dayr al-Qamar (Lebanon)–Biography. |
  Ithaca (N.Y.)–Biography. | Muscular dystrophy–Patients–United
  States–Biography.
Classification: LCC CT275.M18 A3 2017 | DDC 920.72–dc23
LC record available at https://lccn.loc.gov/2017000738

Editing, book design, and composition by Adept Content Solutions, Urbana, IL.

Contents

Prologue

Phoenician stones I touched as a child
Awaken, asking, again and again,
Where have you been all these decades?
Lost, I answer, drowning in waterless pools.

Where have you been? they ask, invading my memory
As mountainous winters covered our old bones with snow.

Where have you been? they ask,
As spring rains prepared us to welcome summer sun.

Your touch so long ago still haunts us,
Your small hands caressing us as you climbed
Stairs too steep for your small feet.

A Street in Deir el-Amar with the Malti house on the left.

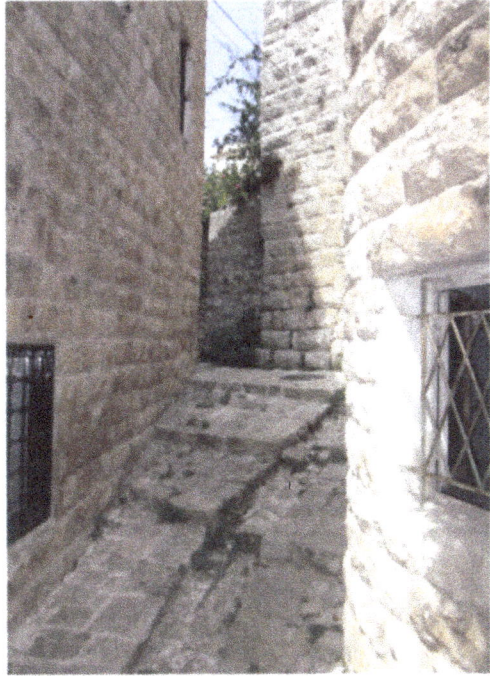

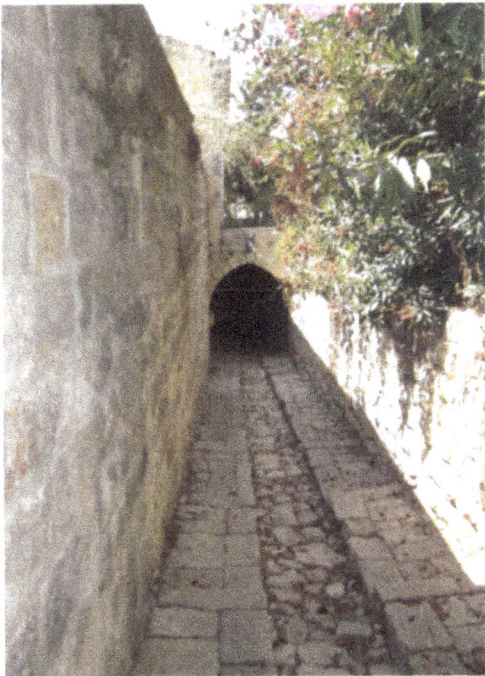

Tunnel leading to St. Elias and the rest of the village.

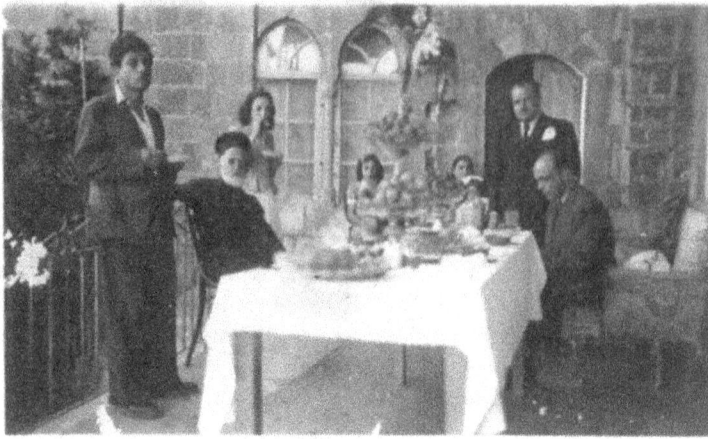

On the balcony with the Melkite priest.
Lemon tree on the left, c. 1953

Odette holding Constantine,
Papa, and Fedwa c. 1948

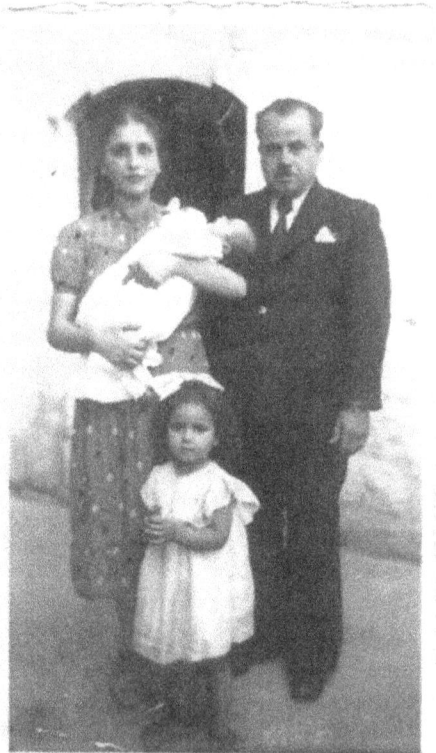

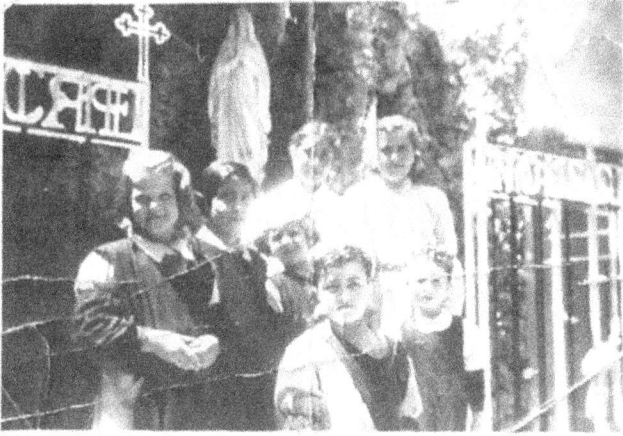

Fedwa and classmates in front of the Grotto

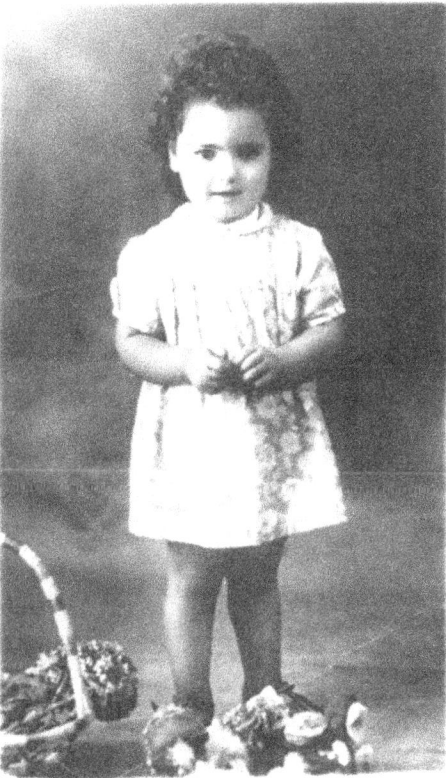

Fedwa in Easter dress,
c. 1951

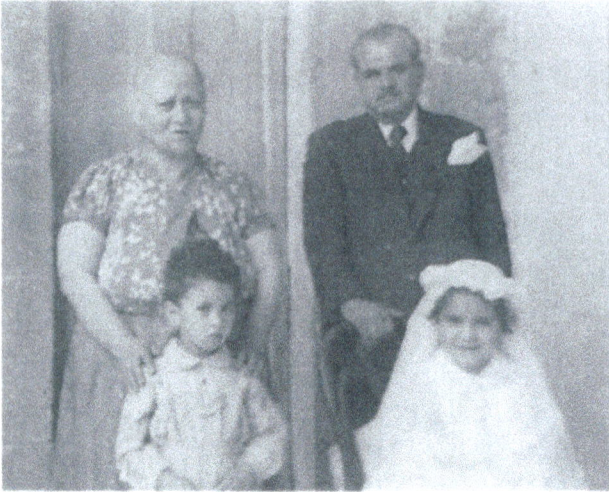

Aunt Najla, Papa, Constantine, and Fedwa in her First Communion dress, c. 1954

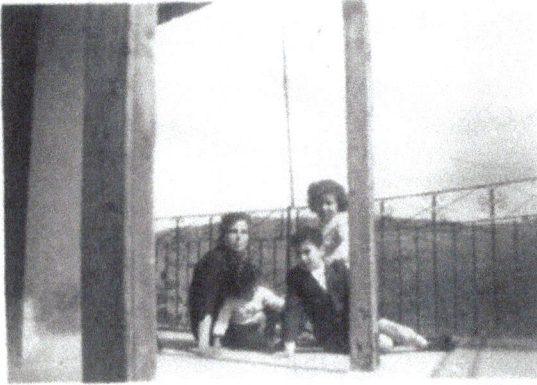

Hana, Mimo, Constantine, and Fedwa on the 3rd floor balcon with Shouf Mountains in the back, c. 1957

My best friend Marie, just before my leaving Lebanon, 1959

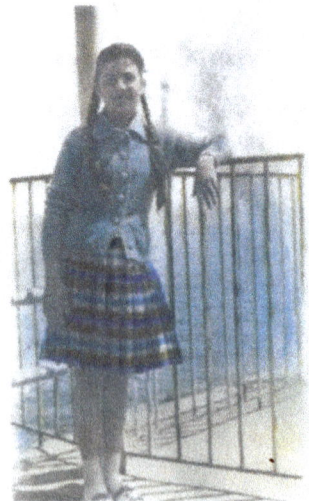

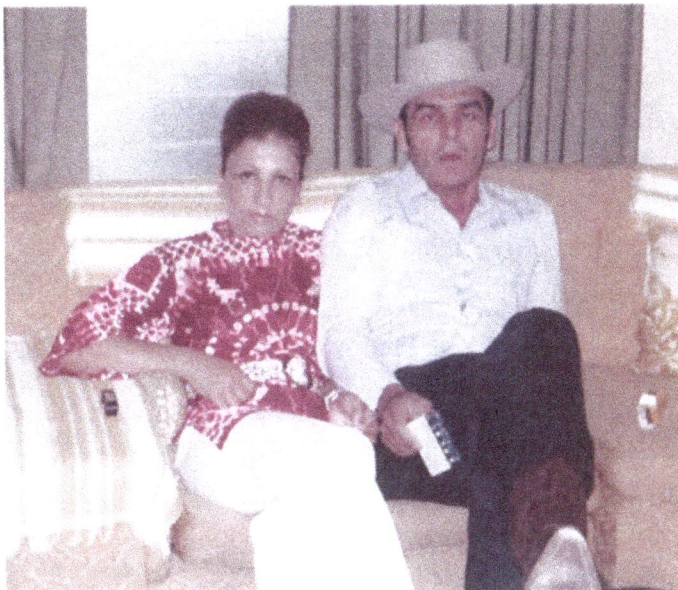

Odette and Joe
in 1973

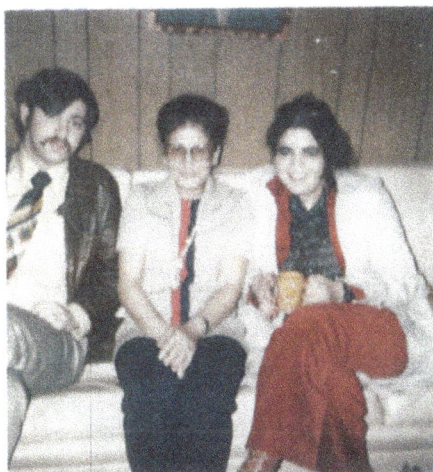

Allen, Odette,
and Fedwa in
Mississippi,
1977

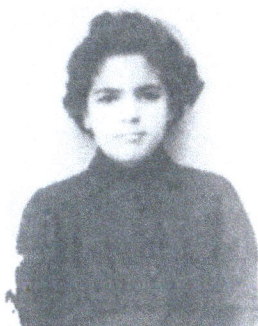

Fedwa's official
identity picture
before leaving
Lebanon, 1959

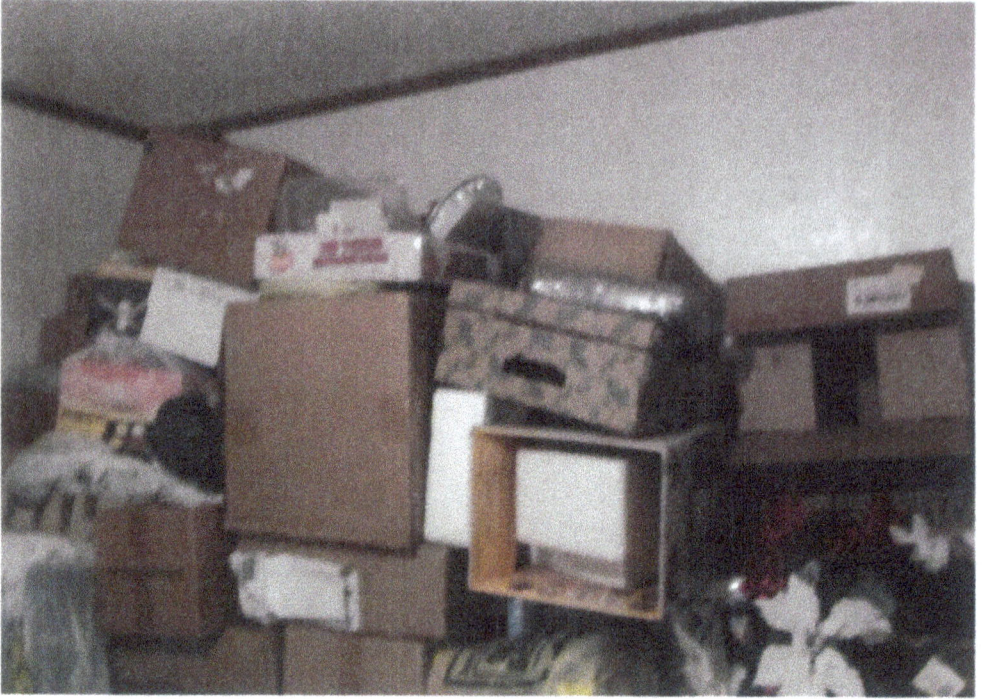

Room in Odette's house, 2012

Odette and
Constantine,
c. 1982

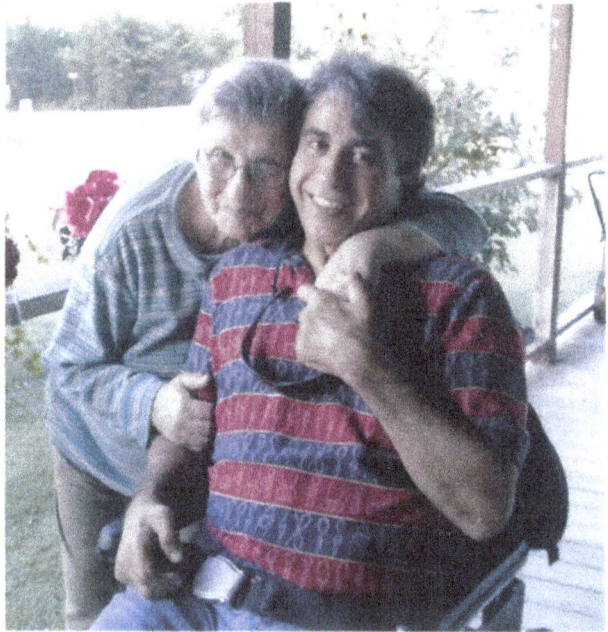

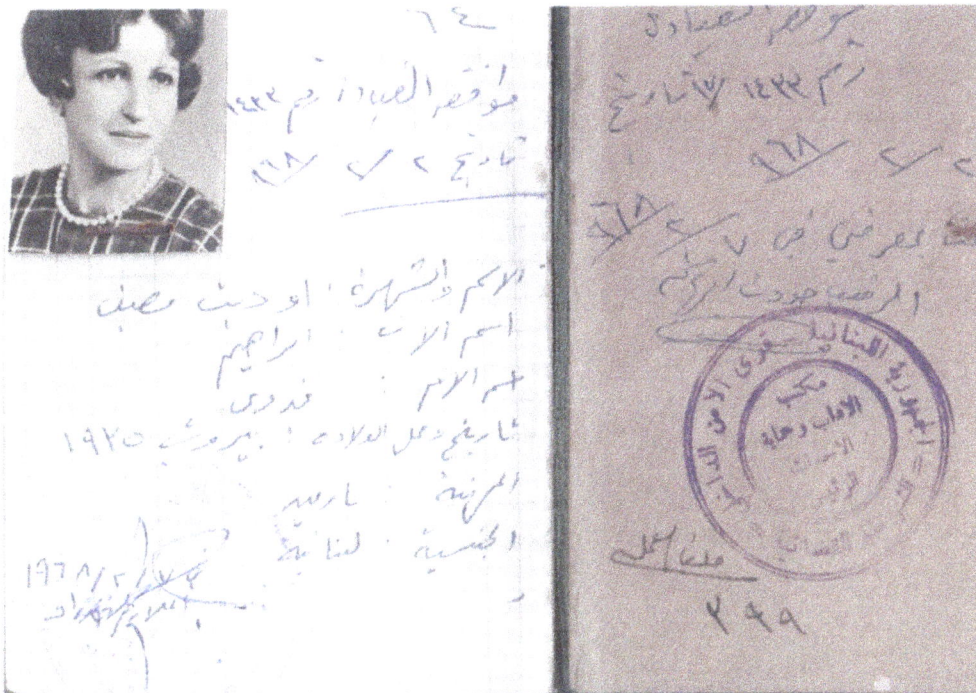

Work Papers, 1968

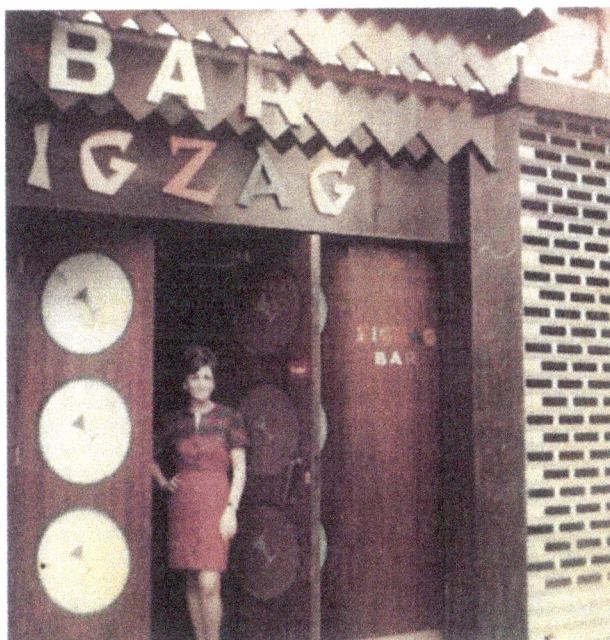

Odette at the
Zigzag Bar,
1968

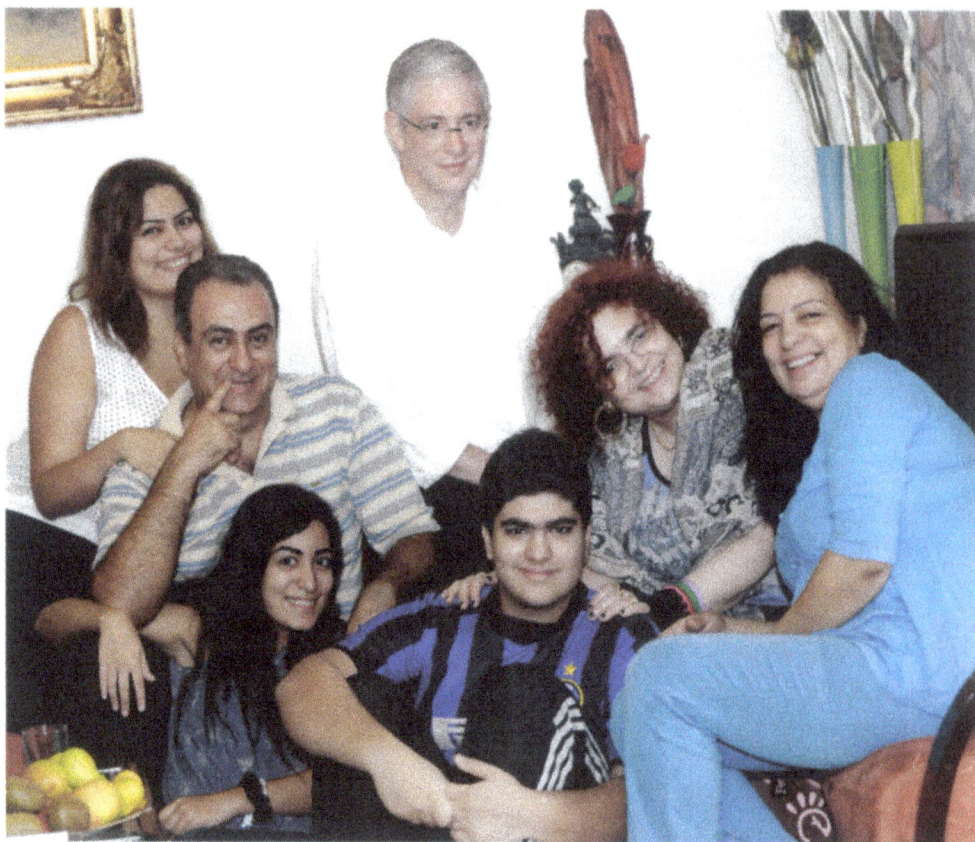

Clockwise from top-left: Rola, Allen, Fedwa,
Mimo, Imad, Yara, and Halim, 2010

PART I
Albert

CHAPTER 1

Abode of the Moon

Nothing could match the location of the Malti house in Deir el-Amar (the Abode of the Moon). One of the most famous villages in Lebanon, Deir el-Amar is nestled in the Shouf Mountains, about a two-hour drive from Beirut on winding mountain roads, which cars shared with meandering sheep. Steeped in the country's tumultuous history and boasting Ottoman palaces, Deir el-Amar was a stop on the road to Beit el-Din. There, a preserved Ottoman palace serves as the summer residence of the president of Lebanon, where he can exchange the Beirut heat for the cool breezes of the Shouf Mountains.

Two churches flanked our three-story family house in Deir el-Amar. One church, up a steep set of enormous stairs, was visible from the back kitchen window of our third floor. The other, St. Elias, was a large complex that enclosed a church, a seminary, and living quarters for priests and visiting dignitaries.

One entered our house through a large metal double door, leading into an even larger rectangular courtyard. To the left and down some stairs, the visitor encountered another courtyard. This one was square, with a living room/salon facing the stairs and my father's medical clinic to the left. At the end of the courtyard was a Turkish toilet (a hole in the floor over which one squats). Occupying the place of honor was an enormous lemon tree whose buds perfumed the entire house in springtime. The tree stood tall, as if proud of its status as the closest neighbor of my father's clinic, over whose entrance it hovered like a mother over her child. When I was little, I was sure that if the tree chose to speak, it would reveal timeless secrets.

Inside Papa's clinic, a large desk faced a window with a view of the courtyard and the lemon tree. Thick medical books and stacks of journals inhabited the top of the desk, and a large wooden swivel chair accompanied it. The clinic also boasted a glass-top table on wheels with medical instruments and vials of liquids unfamiliar to me, as well as chairs reserved for the physician and patients. Another table held medical pamphlets and fliers. A covered bench, tucked into a recess in the left wall, served those who needed to lie down for Papa's examination.

The living room was a mass of intricately woven and colorful Oriental wool carpets. More a salon in the Middle Eastern fashion than a Western parlor, it boasted a high sitting area with woolen cushions. Oriental carpets covered the floor. In the back corner, a piano concealed its existence, since my Aunt Najla, once a talented piano player, was now too crippled to approach her favored instrument. Behind the piano, a curtain opened to reveal another set of stairs, at the bottom of which rested the old Ford that Papa no longer drove. Keeping the car company were enormous glass barrels of freshly pressed olive oil from our olive groves. Opposite the car and the olive oil, in the same oversized hallway, a permanently locked door led to the world outside the family home.

This salon was at once public and private. It was where the Malti family entertained guests, served the legendary Easter feast, and celebrated the Christmas holiday. But it was also where our live-in companion slept: an old, almost-deaf woman, Umm Zahiyya. My brother Constantine (Qustantine in Arabic, and hence the nickname Costy) and I sometimes joined her for the night, cuddling with our cats on the Oriental carpets.

On the other side of the lemon tree, a long flight of stairs led to the uppermost floor of the house, which was surrounded by a kind of veranda we called the *balcon*. There was nothing more wonderful than the *balcon* in summer, when mattresses appeared as if by sleight-of-hand on its floor. We slept in the open air, gazing at the star-studded sky, and the entire village seemed to live outdoors.

Our *balcon* vied with Aunt Najla's roof for pleasure on summer nights. It was on those nights that we village children contributed to transforming the roofs from open-air sleeping places to spots where people spent more time awake than asleep. Summer nights became festivals of singing and playing: conversations between neighbors, children yelling at their friends, balls thrown in games of catch from roof to roof, and songs reaching into the air.

The top-floor *balcon* was also where my father, quite the marksman, stood to hunt birds in flight. One summer day, he shot a long snake that had terrified us as it slithered around the base of the lemon tree. His master bedroom with wonderful Ottoman arched doors and windows adjoined the *balcon*, as did four other bedrooms. To the side of the master bedroom were a kitchen and a bathroom replete with a shower and a toilet (yes, the Turkish kind).

The bottom floor with the clinic and salon, along with the top floor, boasting the *balcon* and bedrooms, constituted one side of the house. The other side, at a level situated between the two floors and separated from them by the enormous entranceway, was Aunt Najla's domain. It extended from her large bedroom/

salon with three doors, one of which led to an equally large storage room with stacked boxes and trunks against the back wall and locked metal closets on the side wall shared with the bedroom. For me as a child, the locked closets were a mystery, and I stared at them every time I passed by.

The two residential areas, that of my father and that of Aunt Najla, were surrounded by a yard with a garden and a mammoth fig tree. The fig tree had been grafted to bring forth a variety of figs. No matter what the size or shape, the fruit of that tree tasted of Paradise: fleshy, sweet like honey, with minute seeds, all enveloped in a soft skin that varied from green through purple to black in different combinations and shades.

In that yard, the woman who helped her husband take care of our family farm arrived at dawn to bake fresh bread. I always awoke early to watch her. An overweight, elderly matron with hair wrapped in a colorful scarf tied at the back of her head, she sat on the ground in front of the oven, barefoot and cross-legged with her dress drawn up to her knees. The oven's hemispherical top drew its heat from the burning coals below. The woman's hands kneaded the dough and stretched it. An incredibly complicated and graceful dance followed as her hands threw the dough in the air, performing an elegant twist, and then grabbed it as it landed, stretching it a little, and then seducing it into a continuous dance until its thin body was gently laid on the hot oven. When the bread offered itself, it was a veritable delicacy, at once warm and soft but for a slight crunch at its lightly charred edges.

Every morning when I was home from boarding school, I went to the chicken coop next to the fig tree to retrieve fresh eggs to eat for breakfast with the just-baked bread. The chickens sat on shelves atop the straw, hiding their treasures from any intruders while watching the rooster spread his wings, displaying his body as if for battle at the entrance of the coop. His loud shrieks expressed his objections to my act of violation. For me, acquiring the eggs was reminiscent of an obstacle course, but for Costy, it was a battle. When my brother invaded his territory, the rooster would jump on his head and attempt to pluck out his eyes, so Costy learned to protect himself while collecting the prize.

In the space extending from the house entrance and reaching outside and around my aunt's room, there was a cement bench attached to the wall. Past the stairs leading to our salon and the clinic, an open entrance area served for washing laundry and making fresh soap. The farmer's wife and Umm Zahiyya were in charge. They both wore long, embroidered dresses and colorful cotton scarves covering graying hair tied in knots behind their heads, but our live-in companion was tall and thin, whereas the farmer's wife was short and heavy. I remember their faces, warm and friendly, as they talked and laughed, turning a necessary task into a joyous occasion. Even Aunt Najla joined in the gossip and festivities as she sat in a chair and watched the soap-making process.

The two women stood while stirring, with long, unwieldy instruments, a deep cauldron filled with, among other things, gallons of Malti family olive oil. My fascination always led me to walk around the cauldron. Though its height prevented me from seeing the innermost transformations of its contents, it could not stop me from inhaling the wonderful smell of the heated olive oil emanating from its open top. Once the mixture solidified, it was time to cut the soap into uneven white squares, leaving soap shreds lying about.

Cleaning the ground followed the soap making, the running water flowed freely around everyone's bare feet accompanied by our gleeful laughter as our clothing became drenched. The two major actors in this drama, the soap-makers, stood and lifted their wet, long dresses above their knees and then bent down and grabbed the loose material, gathering it tightly to one side of their bodies and wringing out the excess water. They continued squeezing, as the formerly soaked material grew thinner and thinner with each twist until not a drop of water remained.

***

My aunt could not navigate stairs. Hence, her physical world was confined to the middle section of the house, where she ate, drank, and slept. This was also where she performed her bodily functions—a portable metallic bedpan being an essential part of her room. Aunt Najla, for as long as I remember, looked the same: a round face, gray hair tied back behind her head, and a heavy body with sagging breasts. She made all her own clothing, including her undergarments. She never left the house.

When I watched Aunt Najla walk, with her slow, slightly shuffling gait, I was mesmerized by the way her upper calves merged with her lower thighs, in the process swallowing her knees, which, for me, never existed. Now that I am older and living with an inherited form of muscular dystrophy, Charcot-Marie-Tooth disease (I was diagnosed in my early thirties), I look at the back of my legs in the mirror and see those of Aunt Najla. She never spoke of her affliction. I suspect, however, that she must have known of it. Whatever the enigmas in her body, they accompanied her to the grave. As a child, I knew only that Aunt Najla was confined to her part of the house.

Our family was an odd one. Aunt Najla had been trained as a schoolteacher. She was trilingual (Arabic, French, and English), yet, somewhere along the line, she decided not to pursue her own career but to devote herself to her brother, my father. His two marriages, the first to my mother Odette, the second to my stepmother Hana, did not deter Najla from her mission. That brother-sister attachment is not unusual in Arab society.

My paternal grandmother's sister, my father's aunt (I am ashamed to admit that I do not remember her name), was present during my early childhood. She was bedridden and slept in Aunt Najla's room on a floor mattress. I would see her emaciated face on the floor to the right as I entered my aunt's room. High up on the wall near the foot of her bed was an oil lamp to keep the room lit on dark winter nights. My great aunt had visions of Christ, who had appeared to her on the opposite wall, above Aunt Najla's bed. Sometimes I entered that room and sat next to her on the floor, gazing at her wizened face and holding her thin hands. Did she ever speak to me? She may have. I do not remember. I do remember that she spoke to God. For years, I wanted to have visions. After my father died, I prayed that he would appear to me like Jesus had appeared to my great aunt. He never did. I was at once anxious for the visions but also frightened about them. What would I say? What would I do? I did not want to be alone when they occurred.

Aunt Najla was the source of family history. She told me how my grandfather George, the Ottoman medical officer, died. It was during the First World War—by ministering to rat-infested wagons of soldiers. She told me how her sister died: falling as a young girl while walking along the top edge of the high wall that separated our property from that of the neighbors below. She told me about my uncle Constantine the dentist, who also died at a young age. He was an artist of sorts—his calligraphic painting of a bird hung permanently in the family salon. And she told me how awful my mother Odette was.

***

Summer in the village was a precious time. In the late afternoon but long before dark, as the hot sun wound its way toward the horizon, Costy and I would pick fresh figs and apricots from our family orchards. The first pickings of ripe fruit always landed in our mouths, overwhelming our senses with complex tastes. Our urges satisfied, we then placed the ripe fruit in tall wicker baskets with handles. Visiting the family farm in summer was an activity Costy and I shared with Papa. My father would walk, one of his hands holding one of mine, the other one of

Costy's. He took long steps while Costy and I skipped along. We followed paths that wound through bushes, wild herbs, and flowers, elated by the fragrance of wild thyme and other herbs wafting through the air.

Though we did not have a telephone and could not instantly communicate with our farm caretakers, they always seemed to sense our arrival, greeting us with freshly baked bread spread with freshly-churned butter and sprinkled with sugar. The adults sat and talked while my brother and I played with the farmer's children. Surrounding the farmhouse were fields of fruit trees, including persimmons, pomegranates, and oranges—not to mention the usual fig and apricot trees. Visits to the farm were an orgy of the senses: smells and tastes mixing with sight and touch, of taking apart a pomegranate, for example, and freeing its ruby-red seeds from the thin, white veil of skin.

In the evenings, my father liked to climb the long, steep stairs leading to the small church we could see from the kitchen window (not Saint Elias, but another church whose name is lost to memory). Costy and I often joined him, and the three of us would enter the always-open church, dip our fingers in holy water, and cross ourselves in the Eastern way, with the thumb and its adjoining two fingers moving from the forehead to the chest and then to the right shoulder and the left shoulder, before returning to the chest (as opposed to the Catholic way with full right hand moving from the forehead to the chest but going to the left shoulder first and then to the right one and finally to the chest). After saying short prayers, we continued climbing the streets behind the church, making our way uphill on the path that eventually gave out on the main street of the village. As Papa watched for cars, we would cross the road and enter the pastry shop. I always ordered my favorite pastry: two rectangular thin layers of dough dipped in hot oil, their crisp edges surrounding a softer middle, which in turn enveloped a beige, slightly nutty paste whose taste remains with me to this day. As I crunched into the crisp outer layer, the filling sometimes attempted an escape. But I was always vigilant and captured it. Costy loved ice cream (and still does) and would leave the shop, holding in his little hands a rectangular cone surrounding the fragile ice cream coated with bits of fresh pistachio.

***

My father, Albert, studied medicine in Paris and was attached to the famous Hôpital Laënnec. He had a medical practice in Beirut but always kept a clinic in our house in Deir el-Amar, where he would see patients a few days a week. A thoracic specialist, he wrote books about the noxious effects of smoking, yet he smoked heavily.

I was in the habit of entering Papa's clinic when no patients occupied it. When I did not want to be a nun, I wanted to be a physician. One of my favorite childhood books was a biography of Marie Curie. How romantic and exciting her life seemed, working in the laboratory with her husband, Pierre. Years later, when I was inducted into the American Philosophical Society and learned that Marie Curie had been a member, it felt like the fulfillment of a childhood dream.

In addition to the medical books and fliers, the clinic boasted high on one wall a closet whose door reached to the arched ceiling and which contained classics of French literature. Often, I would ask my father to take one down for me: *Le Cid*, Ronsard, and so many others. French culture extended to the medical: brochures featuring pictures of nuns in the French colonies, sent to minister to the sick, sat next to colorful booklets enticing the patient to fantasize about locations in France, like Vichy, to which one could retreat for health reasons and "take the waters."

A medicinal smell greeted me as I entered the clinic. A climb onto my father's chair followed, as with great effort I raised one leg then the other onto the constantly swiveling leather seat. Finally, I could rest my body on the chair, legs dangling, hands barely reaching the desk.

On that desk, a mysterious book awaited me: enormous, bound in reddish-brown leather. My hands moved, as though independent of my body, toward the thick volume. Slowly, slowly, my right fingers would turn the pages. In the middle of the book were heavy plastic sheets that seemed proud of their difference from the other pages around them. Each sheet had its own colorful illustrations. Two or three sheets could be laid one on top of the other to generate different forms and shapes alien to my young eyes.

Too young to understand the massive book, I appreciated its beauty. If Papa entered the room, I would ask him to identify the colorful shapes for me. He named body parts. Ah! Body parts. I imagined that my own small body was full of such wonders. I knew I had a stomach but had no idea it could be so colorful. I could spend hours in Papa's chair as my eyes gobbled up the shapes and colors of the heavy see-through plastic pages. It was magic. Flip one sheet and the shapes and colors changed. Flip another and yet more shapes and colors appeared. Nothing can come close to my childhood companion. True, contemporary anatomy books have similar plastic pages, but their pages cannot recreate the irreplaceable rainbows of that lost time. What happened to Papa's anatomy book with its dazzling pages? I have no idea. All I know is that it left my world—like the past, like my father.

***

It was the Easter holiday, and I was home from boarding school. I was seven or eight years old. The sun was shining as I looked out from the third-floor enormous *balcon* and saw houses below, descending into a valley rich with greenery. The valley turned into a hillside of rising terraces laden with blooming fruit and wide olive trees. I held on to the wrought iron fence. I was short and could barely reach the top, but I could see the cars winding their way on the curving road to the palace of Beit el-Din. I knew it well. My grandfather, a medical officer in the Ottoman army, tended to the palace and its occupants. My father and all his siblings were born in that palace, in a room overlooking the famous square, which boasts in its center a fountain with colorful inlaid tile. Costy and I accompanied Papa on numerous pilgrimages to this sacred spot.

If I made a left turn on the Malti house's third-floor *balcon* surrounding the multiple rooms, I could reach the outside wall of the house. I was able to bring my imaginary telescope closer and concentrate on the towering building a small distance from ours. It was the Melkite Catholic seminary attached to the Church of St. Elias. I called out to Constantine, who quickly arrived, sporting the shorts and shirt that little French boys wear. It was time to watch the seminarians enjoying an afternoon stroll across the roof of their building. We were both fascinated by these young men in their long, black robes, sporting thick, black ribbons around their waists that almost fell to the ground. As the seminarians took their slow steps, the robes moved in the afternoon breeze, and the black ribbons flew in the air behind them. Some walked with their heads down as though in a state of deep spiritual contemplation; others chose to walk, chatting with one of their fellows. They could easily turn around and see those two curious children eagerly following their every move, but they were engrossed in their own world and would return to the seminary, leaving us still staring.

Easter weekend began with a village festival in which both adults and children participated. Costy and I rushed to the Church of St. Elias early in the afternoon to join the fun. We entered the gigantic church courtyard through a set of heavy wooden doors. Linked to the massive church, attached buildings embraced the courtyard with their gray-and-ochre stones. To the left was a building that housed the priest and his wife (priests of the Eastern rite could marry). A back room constituted the priest's office and boasted a large desk and a chair. The prized feature of the office was the telephone, still rare in the village during my childhood. In the salon, the priest's wife offered lucky guests fresh pastries and warm drinks like coffee, *yansoon* (a warm anise drink), or tea. To the right of the courtyard, across from the church, stood the door to a room to which we rushed to retrieve the supplies that would permit us to enjoy our Easter weekend.

Soon, the sound of village footwear created a symphony in the church square: simple clog-like slippers, thick wooden soles with a single leather strap across the toes. Click, clack, clank, clonk: the tone of the wood as it kisses the stone depended on the weight of the individual. A heavier body produced louder bangs when its feet landed one after another on the stone as if the body were playing a drum. The noisy clogs were soon shed. The heat of the ground pounded by the sun was quickly relieved as water flowed freely out of hoses and crashed from full pails. The repeated swishing of tall brooms joined the water music as bristles performed a back-and-forth massage of the pavement. Women and children screaming with joy and laughter provided the chorus. The women directed the broom handles in a dance while we children grabbed the hoses and pointed them at one another, soaking our clothing. All this went on while other church members meticulously cleaned the inside of the sanctuary.

When the sun finally rose on Easter Sunday, church bells resounded throughout the village as people entered the Church of St. Elias in newly purchased clothing. All children received new spring outfits for Easter, and it was a ritual for all the neighbors to compliment one another's offspring as they offered holiday greetings. Papa, each hand in one of ours, guided us to a front pew. Young priests welcomed us as they walked through the aisles. Incense burners flew on long triple chains held by their swinging arms. Smoke, escaping the golden orbs, enveloped us in its heavenly cloud. I was intoxicated during the mass when I sat next to Papa. I tell myself it was the incense combined with the music, the singing, and the pageantry.

After Easter Mass, we returned home, jumping and running, while Papa was busy chatting with friends and neighbors. Afterward, he would make his normal Sunday rounds from church to church to deliver holiday wishes from the entire Malti family. In our village, the Easter holiday belonged to the Malti family. In a few hours, our gargantuan living-dining room would be filled with guests from various churches, the table overflowing with food: fresh yogurt covered with equally fresh mint from our farm, just-baked bread, assorted stuffed vegetables, fried eggplant, roasted lamb, chicken sitting atop platters of spiced rice with pine nuts, and other delicacies. The highest-quality *arak* (the Lebanese anise-based alcoholic drink, similar to *ouzo*) graced the dining table, along with fresh water and ice for those guests who preferred to add these to their *arak*, transforming it from a clear to a milky white liquid. Candles were lit in the heavy silver candelabras, and after the feast, everyone would relax on backless couches covered with Oriental carpets, drinking Turkish coffee and savoring Lebanese pastries.

CHAPTER 2

City Life and Village Life

My father owned property in Beirut, part of which he used for his medical practice. He regularly drove from the mountains to the seaside capital and often allowed me to accompany him. I loved the drive as much as being in the capital. At times, Papa would stop when he spotted a farmer standing on the roadside, his hands waving items for sale: freshly plucked green chickpeas, still attached to their branches. Papa always handed me the bouquet, and I would entertain myself during the trip eating one fresh chickpea after another, each small, soft pea bursting in my mouth, enveloping it in a taste and texture I cannot begin to describe. Despite the seductive appeal of the fresh chickpeas, I never allowed my eyes to be diverted from the changing scenery as we passed hillside terraces thick with fruit trees, pine, and here and there a cold mountain stream.

If Papa was thirsty, he would stop on the road and walk to a stream, cup his hands in the water to capture some of the cold liquid, and drink it. He taught me to imitate him. Standing legs slightly apart, I had to bend over, my hands approaching the stream flowing down the side of the mountain. Once the limpid water touched my tongue, I could begin to straighten up and swallow the liquid treat. Papa, much more experienced, performed this operation effortlessly. After numerous stops at mountain streams, I too reached a level of mastery.

I never ceased to be amazed how descending the narrow asphalt roads of the Shouf Mountains led to a lively city beside the blue waters of the Mediterranean. My panoramic world morphed drastically as Papa navigated busy city streets between tall buildings. I watched as people fearlessly slid between moving cars, whose horns emitted a variety of noises that blended with the shouts of angry drivers and screeching car brakes. Instead of the familiar music of village church bells, my ears became the repository of a grating symphony of city noises—music composed, it seemed, by a tone-deaf musician.

It did not take me long to realize that the world was much larger than my village, and it did not take me long to love Beirut as much as I loved Deir el-Amar. One place I never tired of in Beirut was Papa's clinic. To my child's eyes, that clinic was enormous. Consultation rooms lined a long hallway. Papa's medical office was in the corner of the building, with windows looking out on the Beirut skyline. It was there that he would place me while he kept busy in the individual treatment rooms.

But I never lacked for attention. Often, the patients were Papa's friends or acquaintances, and they would stop and hug me as they entered and exited the clinic. Then there was always my mother Odette's aunt, a nurse and Papa's clinical assistant, who watched me out of the corner of her eye as I made myself comfortable on the Oriental carpets spread out on Papa's office floor. Odette's aunt had been responsible for my father's marriage to my mother, having introduced her niece, Odette, also a nurse, to the successful respiratory specialist whose practice was her life.

Shortly after his marriage, Papa decided that his new family should settle in the enormous Malti village home, and Odette, a beautiful young woman from the capital, found herself suddenly transplanted to a mountain village. She wore makeup and polished her fingernails, practices both alien and distasteful to her husband's female relatives in Deir el-Amar. My paternal aunt Najla may well have studied in Beirut and become trilingual, but she was accustomed to a simple village life, and kept her body devoid of artificial embellishment.

I always preferred accompanying Papa to Beirut rather than remaining at home in the mountains, because at home, I had to witness dreadful fights between Aunt Najla and my mother. These were not just simple verbal exchanges. They were virtual battles, with each soldier wielding one long broom. The two female combatants started from fixed positions: Aunt Najla at her kingdom door that opened to the enormous entrance courtyard to the house, Odette half-way down the stairs leading from the third floor to the same courtyard.

The marital lodgings were on the third floor, a space Aunt Najla could not access because of the steep stairs leading to it. At first, the enemies approached each other with angry voices, Aunt Najla slowly reaching the bottom of the stairs as Odette descended them. Eventually, their words became screams as they came face to face. Each broom rose slowly as each female body lifted an arm, swinging her broom toward the enemy and finally hitting her. The syncopated thuds of the brooms as they landed on shoulders and backs vied with the screams of the two women.

I always seemed to have a sixth sense about when a battle was brewing. At the first moment of an onslaught, I would run through the kitchen door adjacent to Aunt Najla's room where packages of Lebanese biscuits, a kind of anise-flavored shortbread, lay hidden in the bottom drawer of a cabinet. I would grab a package and run downstairs, hiding myself in a corner between the lemon tree and the door of Papa's clinic, where I would remain, under the illusion that I had somehow become invisible. I would open the package as quietly as I could, seize one, and push it into my mouth, chewing only enough to swallow it. As soon as one cookie was about to disappear, my hand would reach inside the package and grab another. This frenzy of grabbing and stuffing increased in intensity as the screams and broom battles got louder. No matter how much those anise treats distracted my taste buds, the constant one-way trips between the package and my mouth never succeeded in silencing the noises of the war raging above my head. No winner emerged from these battles, which always left me in tears.

Despite their association with these painful childhood moments, throughout my life, I never ceased searching for these anise delicacies. From America to France, from Syria to Morocco, from Egypt to Wales: no matter where I landed in the world, I entered shops and searched, like a woman possessed, for anything that resembled those childhood treats. Many were the times that packages beckoned, and I took them home, only to be disappointed as soon as I opened one and smelled its contents. Finally, I told myself that perhaps those Lebanese anise specialties were the product of an imagination that was always trying to glue back together the pieces of a broken life.

But then one day, and completely unexpectedly, fantasy became reality. My husband Allen (we were married in 1971) and I were living in Tunis on a Fulbright fellowship and house-sitting a US embassy home whose resident had a small dog, Molly. Our task was to take care of Molly, an adorable little pooch, and we walked her every day up and down the residential streets of the Menzah district. On one of these regular excursions, we happened completely by chance upon a grocery store where I felt an irrational pull toward the cookie section. I looked around and almost screamed in shock. There, right in front of me, was a package of my childhood anise biscuits. We bought them, and I immediately opened the package. The cellophane crinkled as I tore it open, and before I realized it, I found myself back in our village home in Deir el-Amar, hiding near the lemon tree, listening to the screams above me. I bit into the object of my longing, and it was as if some secret force, some genie from the *Arabian Nights*, had transported the very treat I had so eagerly chewed as a child across time and space.

CHAPTER 3

St. Joseph

One day, my mother was living in our village home, and the next, she was not. No one offered me an explanation, and there were no goodbyes. All I knew was that I no longer had to live through the terrifying clashes between her and Aunt Najla. What time of year was it when Odette, my mother, vanished from my life? I have no idea.

All my life I have tried to understand this chasm, my separation from my mother. Recently, I imagined a missive from my father, now long deceased.

> Letter from My Dead Father
> I am sorry I annulled
> My marriage to your mother,
> But fights she had with others
> Turned the house into war zones.
> How could I as a doctor
> Then dream of healing patients?

***

I was about four years old when Odette left. Papa approached me one day and asked if I would like to go to school. Aunt Najla had taken to reading with me, and I was a fast learner. The idea of school overwhelmed me with excitement. I remember screaming with joy and hugging Papa's legs, the only parts of him I could reach. I remember he lifted me in the air and kissed me. I remember Aunt Najla's proud smiles. I remember my great aunt's sheer pleasure. Fedwa was going to school. Neighbors learned the news. The priest learned the news. Costy learned the news. I became the object of pride for the family and the neighborhood.

Before I knew it, Papa was taking me by the hand, and we were walking past the Church of St. Elias, through the tunnel leading from the church to the open roads of the village. We passed the old Ottoman prison that had been transformed into the village prison. We walked up a steep hill, passing merchants on the left and underground remnants of an Ottoman palace on the right, finally reaching our destination: the boarding school of Les Soeurs de St. Joseph.

The school was a large stone structure set on a mountainside and surrounded by protective walls. The many-storied building contained dormitories, school rooms, a large cloistered courtyard where students played and where both nuns and students took frequent walks, a refectory (or dining hall) for the students, a refectory for the nuns, a store for both nuns and students, administrative offices, and, of course, a church. The church featured carved wooden confessionals and choir stalls, as well as an imposing altar and colorful Stations of the Cross. The school also had elaborate dining and reception rooms with pianos, rooms richly furnished with large padded chairs, couches, and small wooden tables embedded with white mother-of-pearl. Those imposing rooms were the preserve of church dignitaries, officials from the religious order, as well as guests, including family members visiting their children.

My father was at home in every Christian religious establishment in Deir el-Amar. I should not have been surprised that the Mother Superior greeted him warmly and smiled at me as she welcomed me to her office. I sat listening to Papa and the Mother Superior as they planned my future as a boarder. When the Mother Superior asked me what my own wishes were, I surprised myself by the degree of my enthusiasm.

The Mother Superior took Papa and me on a tour of the enormous facility, including the dormitory where I would have my bed and adjoining night table. I noticed the many beds lining the large room as well as the white curtain surrounding what I would later discover was the sleeping quarters of the sister who monitored the students in the dormitory. Papa and I also visited the refectory. Long rectangular wooden tables equipped with equally long benches had drawers every few feet with small round knobs. The Mother Superior explained to Papa and me that each boarder had her designated seat and her own drawer.

***

Life in boarding school was stimulating; it was my first official introduction to both French and Arab cultures. Memorization, dictation, recitation: I was an avid learner and according to school correspondence, always first in my class. Before I became an official boarder, I had to have uniforms: winter ones, summer ones, and ones for the transitional seasons. The winter uniform was an almost-black dark navy, a pleated skirt and a button-down jacket with a collar under which

I wore a white shirt. The summer uniform was a white-and-light-blue checked dress. The other outfit was a jumper under which one wore a blouse. All this new clothing reached the knee and was complemented by knee-high socks and shoes. A village seamstress measured me, and I became the proud owner of school uniforms that lasted until I outgrew them.

The refectory at Les Soeurs de St. Joseph holds a permanent place in my mind. We students consumed all our daily meals in that grand hall. On one of the walls was a large crucifix, visible from anywhere in the room. To sit at the refectory table involved lifting one leg at a time over the bench so that one's body rested next to the table; only then was it possible to sit down. The supervising nun, in charge of leading us in prayer before the meal, walked back and forth, rosary in hand, one eye on God as she prayed, the other on the sitting students as they ate.

One refectory meal remains particularly alive for me. It contained some kind of sausage. On the surface, the long, circular, brown piece of food bore a distant resemblance to cooked *kofta*. *Kofta* is a typically Lebanese dish made of finely chopped lean lamb meat mixed with diced onion, parsley, and spices, formed into ovals and grilled on skewers. One can consume the grilled *kofta* on its own or in a pita sandwich with pickled vegetables and tahini sauce, or it can be eaten with fresh yogurt and the typical Lebanese rice with bits of fried vermicelli. A more elaborate version of the rice would include pine nuts.

The piece of food facing me that day looked vaguely like a *kofta*, so I grabbed a fork with my left hand and a knife with my right. When I began cutting, I realized it was not soft like *kofta* that could be eaten with the fingers; instead this strange fare sported some kind of see-through outer covering protecting the mixture, through which I realized I had to slice. I cut a piece of the unknown object on my plate and, with great hesitation, placed it in my mouth.

When I bit into what my fork had carried to my mouth, I was sure I was going to vomit. Not only did I have to break the outer covering with my teeth, but the inside seemed a mass of pieces of meat of varied, unsettling textures. The taste was at once unfamiliar and repellent. I held the mixture in my mouth while my right hand traveled to the jacket pocket of my school uniform. I managed to find a little cloth handkerchief (one of many) Aunt Najla had embroidered for me when I went off to live with the nuns. The cloth was still folded. Looking around to make sure that the supervising nun was far away, I took the cloth and placed it on my mouth and nose as though I were about to sneeze, then spat the solid chunk of food into it. Slowly, I opened my personal drawer and shoved the captured object as far back as I could into a corner, making sure it touched the wood, thereby becoming invisible. Then I retrieved Aunt Najla's gift and returned the soiled hankie to its warm place in my pocket.

The next day, during morning recess, a nun summoned me to the Mother Superior's office. Students were called to the Mother Superior's office if they had a visitor or if they had committed an infraction. I gladly accompanied the nun, thinking Papa must be paying me a visit. But no. As soon as I entered the office, I spotted a dried piece of food sitting on a plate glaring at me accusingly.

"Fedwa, do you recognize this object?" asked the Mother Superior with a stern voice, looking me in the eyes.

I was silent.

"You don't have to answer," continued the head of the school, her voice even more stern. "Sister B. found it in your refectory drawer. Would you like to say anything?"

I was still silent. But now I was looking at the floor, a sign that I am sure the Mother Superior correctly interpreted as guilt.

Unsure how to respond, I decided to say nothing.

"All right," said the Mother Superior, "you will be locked in the punishment room until Sister B. comes to get you for dinner. If you need to use a bathroom, you can knock on the door, and someone will accompany you and bring you back. I will also call Dr. Albert to let him know" (meaning my father. In the Middle East, one normally uses someone's first name with their title).

Not a word escaped my mouth. I was deeply ashamed and allowed Sister B. to take me by the hand and guide me to the punishment room. I stepped into the space and heard the door being locked from the outside. To call this area a "room" was an exaggeration. It was even smaller than a typical American toilet at a roadside gas station, which normally includes a sink. The little space in which I found myself alone had no such amenity. There was a small step just inside the door of the "punishment room" which led to a dark wooden bench. I climbed the step and sat on the bench. I looked around the barren space and realized that its walls and ceiling were also made of dark wood. There was no window and no light.

The time alone in the dark was an effective penalty. I thought it harsh as a child, but at the same time, I recognized that I had done something I should not have. Papa had never laid a hand on me or Costy. He may even have been a bit too lenient. The only time he showed any frustration toward me was when I refused to eat a dinner he had cooked. His response was simple. I had to forego the meal, which I happily did.

Sitting alone in the dark allowed my mind to wander. I began by reciting various pieces of literature I had memorized in boarding school. Then I sang songs. But what most entertained me was making up stories. I started with my co-boarders. What were their families like? Had their mothers disappeared? Did they have brothers and sisters? From my co-boarders, I moved to concocting narratives about relatives I had never met, an infinitely more seductive ground for my imagination. What was my aunt wearing when she took that fatal fall from the top of the wall? What did she look like? Was she enjoying herself, unaware of the danger awaiting her? Where did my uncle Constantine do his drawings? Why was he, a trained dentist, interested in art? How did he die?

The time passed quickly. Sister B. knocked on the door and accompanied me to dinner. I took my seat in silence, conscious of the stares the other boarders directed my way. I was familiar with those stares since I myself had participated in them when other students had been isolated for punishment. They were not looks of derision but ones of curiosity and sympathy. Soon, I would have to reveal to my school friends the reason for my sentence. Some were receptive since they also hated those sausages, and others wished that they could have consumed my long-discarded meal.

I never disposed of food in my drawer again. I became, however, more wary of refectory fare, surreptitiously moving servings around my plate, taking small bites of unfamiliar dishes with great hesitation. If I found a piece of food extremely distasteful, I would play the fake sneezing game and edge that food onto one of Aunt Najla's beautiful handkerchiefs. But instead of emptying the contents of the cloth into the wooden drawer, I would slip the napkin back to its resting place inside my uniform pocket. Then I was at leisure to dispose of the offensive tidbit at some later time.

In the interim, I learned from the boarders that the nuns cleaned out our drawers assiduously after dinner, which accounted for my having had to face the Mother Superior during that morning's recess. Was Papa ever informed of my disgraceful act by the Mother Superior, as she had threatened? I will never know, since my indulgent father never spoke to me of the incident. Perhaps he assumed that my isolation had been sufficient punishment. Besides, had he not left me in the care of Les Soeurs de St. Joseph, who were now responsible not only for my formal education but, perhaps more importantly, for my social and personal skills?

To this day, however, I have trouble eating sausage links, especially if they happen to be a bit on the large side. If I inadvertently take a bite of one, I become immediately nauseated as I travel back in time to those boarding school days. Then I do exactly what I did as a child: I take my napkin to my mouth and spit out the offensive morsel.

***

When I entered Les Soeurs de St. Joseph, I was one of the youngest boarders and shared the dormitory with girls slightly older than I was. We girls thought ourselves fairly ingenious. We had developed a set of nightly activities after we made sure we could hear the nun snoring behind her curtain in the corner. One of the older students convinced us that we could give ourselves a cold with a high temperature if we followed her directions. We simply had to sneak out of the sleeping quarters in the middle of the night and make our way slowly and quietly—if not soundlessly—to the bathroom with its sinks and windows facing the mountains. Then we were to take turns repeatedly hanging our heads out the open windows and breathing in the cold night air. This adventure lasted a good while, since one stop at a window was not enough to guarantee a high temperature.

This game complete, we returned just as silently to our beds, again listening for the nun's snoring. Sleep after such excitement overtook us easily. It always seemed much too early for the nun to ring the bell announcing a new day. She would stand fully dressed at the end of the line of beds, watching us squirming while trying to wake ourselves. Thermometer in hand, she would begin her slow march down the line of beds. Those of us who had performed the nightly experiment raised our hands. The nun then made her way to the individual beds. When she got to me, I would open my mouth, feeling the cold thermometer slip under my tongue. I would hold it until the nun's hand pulled it out.

I always watched in anticipation as the nun's eyes centered on the medical instrument. Disappointment set in when the nun slowly shook her head, a signal that I had no temperature and should begin dressing myself. Too bad. Not a single one of us girls who had ventured in the middle of the night to breathe cold air ever got a temperature. In my more lucid moments, I cannot help but wonder if our supervising nun knew all along what we naïve and foolish little girls were up to in the middle of the night. I suspect she did. Perhaps it is my imagination, but I seem to remember her always with a little smirk as she watched her charges disappointedly readying themselves for the full day ahead.

***

We were all familiar with the bathroom during the daytime. It was there that the nuns washed us down. At the time, there was only cold running water at the boarding school. On cleaning day, we undressed in our dormitory and walked to the bathing room. On the right as one entered were large round metal tubs low on the floor over whose edges we could step. First, we stood naked in the cold. While one nun heated water, the others joined us with a pail in which the hot water had already been mixed with the cold. The nuns would grab a round sponge, rub it in soap, and start washing our little bodies from the top down. During the cold winter in the mountains, we could not help but shiver.

Each of us had nothing better to do than gaze at one another naked, watching our own bodies develop through the eyes of our friends. We knew whose breasts were getting larger over time and whose legs were thicker. We knew who had pubic hair growing. None of this shocked us. Our bodies were visible to everyone around us, including the nuns in charge of washing our most intimate parts. The only sensation I believe any of us ever had was being cold and shivering in consequence. We certainly never felt shame. Unlike other women I know, I am not shocked when seeing naked female bodies or being naked in the company of other women.

I was a little older, perhaps six or seven, when I changed dormitories. There, we did not play night games because we were farther away from the washing room. Every Thursday morning, however, we changed the bed sheets. Because of the refreshing air from the open windows, I suspect I must have moved to that space in the spring. Each of us was given fresh sheets, and we were taught how to remake our beds. Since the boarding school was on a mountainside, I could look out the windows and see the mountains so close by that I could practically touch the trees.

No matter what the dormitory, I was never absent from the schoolrooms for a single day, and this despite the fact that I raised my hand and opened my mouth on more than one morning in excited anticipation that the peripatetic thermometer might, if only once, look kindly upon me and provide me with a high temperature.

***

Education with Les Soeurs de St. Joseph was not solely through the written word. Ballet was on the menu early in our educational training. I confess that I was never very graceful at that. Though I was able to perform in front of the audience of parents and students, I could not keep my body standing on my toes very long. Now that I am more familiar with my physical predicament, I cannot help but wonder if I was displaying the very early, and barely visible, signs of the form of muscular dystrophy that has been passed down, knowingly or not, from one Malti generation to the next.

The French nuns were vigilant about their students' memorization of popular French songs, like:

Auprès de ma blonde, qu'il fait bon, fait bon, fait bon,
Auprès de ma blonde, qu'il fait bon dormir.
(Next to my blond [female], how good it is to sleep)

Not only did we young girls learn verses like these by heart, but we also acted them out on the auditorium stage in the boarding school. Some of the girls played the role of young women, sitting in little boats and wearing white frilly dresses and straw hats with ribbons hanging down their sides, while other girls played sailors, standing in the boats and wearing a dark navy blue-and-white uniform with round sailors' hats with a red pompom on top. The sailors, at the bow and stern of the boats, hands on wooden oars, sang to the smiling girls seated on wooden benches that stretched from port to starboard.

What role did I play? I was one of the sailors whose voice rang out along with those of my cross-dressed female colleagues. Papa always attended these performances and, along with other parents and audience members, proudly clapped in appreciation when we pseudo-French players completed our act.

The sexuality of the tune strikes me only now: the male sailor who repeatedly sings of his desire to sleep alongside his blond girlfriend. What were we young Lebanese girls mimicking? These cross-cultural games never seemed strange to me when I lived in the hermetic atmosphere of a French order of nuns. Here we were: little dark-skinned, dark-haired girls dressed as French sailors singing of their blond girlfriends to other dark-skinned, dark-haired girls dressed in contrasting white frilly dresses. French culture, with all its missionary zeal, was an essential part of the individual I was (and still am) as it was of my father whose medical studies and practice had led him to the French capital. I was growing up multiculturally and multilingually in a country, the majority of whose inhabitants shared my complex identity.

***

Papa faced me, right hand outstretched. I interpreted this as a sign that we were about to leave our home for some unknown location. Papa did not offer any information, nor did I ask. For me, this was normal; most often adults did not provide explanations, only the emotional connection of the physical touch. I stretched out my left hand, grabbing his. It was enormous, enveloping mine. I wanted to say my hand reached my father's waist, but that would be a lie. I was short and curly-haired. Papa appeared enormous to me. His hand was strong, guiding me out of the house, first to the right, past a house on our left, and then up the steep stairs, also on our left—stairs so high I could barely reach from one to the next. Papa's hand helped me climb. The stairs were so wide that each could accommodate two of my bodies lengthwise.

Where were we going? Were it nighttime, I would know. My brother's right hand would be attached to my father's left. There would be a lightness to the six legs floating from step to step, heading for the pastry shop and ice cream store. But no, it was just the two of us, Papa and me, climbing the interminable steps, at the top of which the small church greeted us. As always, we stopped inside for a brief prayer and a blessing. Then we continued past the church, up the hill, and through the narrow, curvy streets protected from the sun by the stone buildings on each side. The thick stones spoke of comfort and security. Eventually, we exited the shadowy world into a large sunny, open square. On our left were little shops, lined up one next to the other, inseparable one from the next. Like Atlas, they held up the famous village coffee shop with its outdoor veranda.

I raised my eyes. Men of different ages sat and smoked cigarettes and *nargilas*, those famous water pipes on the top of which tobacco smoldered and from whose side jutted a small rubber hose with a flat replaceable wooden tip around which the smoker wrapped his lips and inhaled the water-cooled tobacco. I could see mouths moving, sometimes in laughter, sometimes involved in animated conversations whose contents remain secret to me.

I pulled my eyes away as Papa's hand gently pulled me toward a cobbler's shop. Before we entered, Papa stopped to greet the other shopkeepers on the way. I stole a glance through the glass front into the cobbler's shop, where my eyes traveled to the counter behind which the shoemaker sat. He was a thin man, with dark skin, a long waxed black mustache curling up his cheeks, and a leather apron covering the bottom half of his body. A round can of shoe polish rested in his left hand, and a well-worn cloth in his right. The cloth rubbed the polish until the two became one. The cobbler's left hand nimbly moved, abandoning the can and grabbing a shoe. The cloth massaged the leather that expressed its gratitude by showing off a magnificent shine.

My father opened the door to the shop, and the cobbler got up from his seat, wiping his hands on a cloth. The cobbler greeted Dr. Albert and his little daughter. He offered us drinks. His assistant, a young boy, ran out of the shop and returned with Papa's coffee and my lemonade. We sat down, and the shop owner took his place on a low, round stool that swiveled. I was confused, unsure of the reason for this surprise visit. Bits of leather in different shapes and different shades of brown, black, dark green, and maroon littered the floor of the shop. Large rolls of leather hid on shelves embedded in the walls. An intense smell of leather mixed with shoe polish invaded my nostrils.

I overheard a quick conversation between my father and the cobbler. My feet were then measured in myriad ways, including from toes to heel and heel to ankle. Then the cobbler wrapped the supple black leather loosely around my feet and deftly cut the shape for a new pair of shoes. Papa specified the color black to match my school uniform.

Weeks later, we returned to the cobbler. Upon our entering the shop, the cobbler and our preferred drinks greeted us. The new shoes were ready, nestled in the cobbler's hands. They were ankle boots. I was not expecting ankle boots. I blocked the tears struggling to stream out of my eyes. I tried to hide my disappointment. The cobbler paid no attention to my sad face, carefully slipping laces into eyelets. Then he smiled at me. Grabbing my feet one at a time with his skilled hands, he lovingly slipped them into their new home. Then he pulled the laces back and forth until they merged. The hands of the cobbler softly separated the laces, but only briefly, since they would come together into a bow atop my shoes.

I watched each action carefully. My patent leather Mary Janes sat on the side of the counter, ignored. I looked at them sadly, longingly. But there was no time for sentimentality. Papa, anxious to see the results, urged me to get up in my new shoes. I followed his directions. My feet imprisoned, I walked a few steps inside the shop and a few steps outside.

The cobbler had not stopped smiling. He wished me good health with my new shoes, the normal litany for a newly acquired item. Papa seemed pleased. We followed the reverse route home. One of my hands sat inside Papa's hand, the other held desperately onto my Mary Janes, now in a paper bag.

Looking back, it is unclear to me why my memory of these new shoes was so colored with sadness. Weren't these boots simply destined for scouting activities, a part of our school training? Was it that I was not mentally prepared for this less-girlish footwear? Or was it because in my later life, ankle boots, like other sensible shoes, were linked to my muscular dystrophy?

CHAPTER 4

The Smell of Death

Death was a familiar, unthreatening presence in the landscape of my childhood, in part because it was not yet real.

Papa was a frequent visitor to the village cemetery, located on the edge of town where the road began its curved, mountainous descent to the Lebanese capital. The cemetery was on a steep hillside, with the tombstones facing the mountains opposite the burial grounds. On many occasions, I accompanied my father as he held my hand and we made our way alongside the road. The distance from our house to the cemetery was quite far, involving a long walk through the village streets from our home to the main road that cut through Deir el-Amar, a walk followed by the long adventure on the asphalt road leading from the village to Beirut.

The approach to the cemetery itself was a visual feast. My eyes always first encountered the tall trees hovering over the graves, resting in uneven rows on the expansive hillside. Dominating the panoramic view were the crosses atop gravestones.

Papa and I would meander over the uneven ground, encountering here and there colorful wild flowers sprouting from the earth. Many of the tombstones were clearly objects of pride for the families in question: well taken care of, polished stones bearing the names of the departed and fresh flowers adorning the ensemble. Every time Papa passed a cross, he would cross himself, and I, imitating him, would do the same.

The Malti burial spot was hard to miss: a monumental two-sided metal gate with a triangular top on which sat a large metal cross. The gate bearing the Malti name was secured by a heavy metal lock. All the metal was intricate filigree, with the shape of the cross dominating the design.

As a child, I would shove my face against the gate in an attempt to view the inside. Stairs led down from the gate into an enormous crypt below. I could see the bottom of the stairs, next to which was open ground. There was a back wall that seemed to lead further underground. The darkness of the space gave free rein to my imagination. I always wanted to ask Papa if that dark wall I could barely see was actually made up of large coffins placed one atop another. But whenever I turned around to look at Papa, he would be on his knees, eyes closed, hands together in prayer. I would join him.

I confess, however, that mine was a distracted prayer. Unlike Papa, I could not keep my eyes closed. I was fixated on what was hiding behind that metal gate. Whose coffins were resting there? Was my great aunt whom I knew and who had had visions of Christ resting there? Could my dead relatives speak to me? If I opened a coffin, would I see one of my long-gone family members?

When Papa was ready to leave the cemetery, I had to accompany him, but I always did so with disappointment in my heart. As a child, I had irrationally attached myself to my young aunt who had fallen to her death while walking on one of the Malti house walls. Why had she become such an object of fascination for me? I still imagine that I can somehow evoke this long-lost relative. I have no physical evidence of the existence of my father's younger sister. She lives for me only through Aunt Najla's loud screams whenever she discovered that my younger brother and I had walked along the narrow wall over the front door of the house, a wall that brought together the two enormous sides of the Malti home. She lives for me through the fear in those screams.

***

Being a boarder at Les Soeurs de St. Joseph meant that on weekends, I could walk home. Beginning downhill from the boarding school, I skipped down the road through part of a market on my right, allowing me to cross the street and face the town prison. But this was not just any prison. My Aunt Najla, purveyor of local lore, brought historic buildings to life with her stories. The current village prison was an Ottoman structure that had also functioned as a prison when the area was under Ottoman rule. Aunt Najla never hesitated to provide all the gruesome details familiar to the older generation of villagers.

The most direct route to our home passed the prison. The enormous and daunting stone building towering over me had few windows. Legend had it that the Ottomans used to hang live prisoners out of the narrow windows, leaving their bodies to bleed on the rough stone walls until they died. I learned early on in my childhood that if I looked closely as I passed, my eyes could see remnants of the blood stains on the walls.

If I wanted a change of scenery, I could make a left turn on the street facing the prison and head toward the center of the village, dominated by an enormous Ottoman palace. Unlike other Ottoman remnants in the village, but like the prison, this building was well preserved. Enormous wide stairs heralded the entrance to this magical location. I never ceased to be fascinated by the palace whenever I passed it. Aunt Najla had related to me in great detail how one of the Ottoman officials inhabiting that palace had been killed in a particularly gruesome manner. He was dragged out of his quarters and to the street below, down all those numerous steps, by his genitals. She always added that his blood ran down the palace stairs into the street for everyone to see. Obviously, the unfortunate character perished during the experience.

The story of a unique death by dragged genitals, more than the stories of multiple deaths by hanging and bleeding, held endless fascination for me. My childhood imagination tried to reconstruct the event in an effort to understand how it could be possible for people to carry out such an act. As I stood on numerous occasions across the street from the palace staring at those endless steps, I could almost hear the official's death screams.

Well into my scholarly career, I published a study centering on a medieval caliph known for his abilities to uncover criminals and force them to confess. This ruler had no qualms about applying torture and using various cruel physical and mental strategies to extract confessions. I came to look at my childhood fascination with Aunt Najla's story with a different, more critical, eye.

***

Les Soeurs de St. Joseph was where I learned what death supposedly smells like. An enterprising fellow student was behind this discovery. Or, at least, that is what I was told. The knowledge was passed down quasi-secretly. My mentor in this rather strange preoccupation taught me in precise detail how to generate the smell of death:

1. Spread out your hand, preferably the right hand.
   a. Place your four fingers (excluding the thumb) together, and bend them inward toward the palm.
   b. Place the four fingers flat against the palm.
   c. Bend the fingers away from the edge of the palm, so they fold at all three knuckles.
   d. Place the edge of the folded fingers approximately half-way on the palm.
   e. Roll the fingers as far as you can, so they sit almost at an angle against the hand.

     f. Place the thumb atop the rolled fingers. Your nails should be touching
        your palm.

2. The last step consists of pushing the four fingers with the help of the
   thumb against the palm as hard as you can. It was imperative to hold
   this position for at least five minutes, although ten minutes were a better
   guarantee for the desired result: generating the smell of death.

3. Warning: if you do not follow these directions precisely, you are doomed
   to fail.

I abided by my mentor's directions. When it was time to release the fingers from their temporary imprisonment, I learned I must move my palm to my nose as quickly as possible lest any of the odor disappear. Once my palm lay atop my nose, I took a deep breath, inhaling the smell of death.

We students practiced this procedure in small groups or singly. The groups functioned as cheering squads, encouraging the shy among us. Initially, I was one of those reluctant to become involved, and when one of my co-boarders asked me why, I was speechless. Instead of answering, I imitated my peers. Rather than experiencing death, however, we were like knights on a quest for its odor. I confess that the reasons for my initial hesitation might have seemed mere superstition. Might I be inviting death into my life and that of my family by creating its smell and, by extension, its presence? Shamed into doing what my young friends were at ease doing, I suddenly smelled death. My palm emitted a strange but complex odor: a musty smell of something that had not seen the open air for a long time, a strong smell of old dirty sheets, a smell that reminded me of my bedridden great aunt, whose position on her floor mattress never changed.

Once I naively became comfortable with the notion that one could generate the smell of death, I would do it at odd times whenever I was alone. Those steps that had seemed so complicated became simple and quasi-automatic. To this day, I clutch my fingers in my palm in an effort to recreate that bizarre odor. At the same time, I wonder how it was that we young girls were so enamored by the smell of death when we should have been searching for the smell of life.

CHAPTER 5

Coming of Age

I first met St. Bernadette in Papa's clinic. She introduced herself to me through the French pamphlets encouraging pilgrimages to Lourdes and touting the miraculous powers of that site, especially the famous grotto that is now permanently installed in my brain. I read and reread the story of Bernadette and dreamed that someday I might travel to Lourdes and see the Virgin myself.

One day, I was awakened in boarding school in Deir el-Amar by a nun, informing me that the Mother Superior wished to see me. The nun accompanied me while I walked slowly, trying to remember anything I could have done to deserve what would surely be a severe punishment. Instead, a smiling Mother Superior ushered me into her office. I became more and more anxious. Oddly, the Mother Superior was fully relaxed as she informed me that my school performance was excellent and that she and the other nuns were very proud of me.

My mind began to wander when I suddenly heard the name "Bernadette."

"What?" I asked the Mother Superior.

"Your father, Dr. Albert, donated money to our school to build an exact replica of the grotto with St. Bernardette and the Holy Virgin at Lourdes."

I was speechless. An ever more enormous smile spread across the Mother Superior's face as she informed me that Papa was coming to the boarding school that very day, when an official unveiling of the newly-built monument was to take place. My curiosity was overwhelming. But I was not quite sure what to ask the Mother Superior. Papa had revealed nothing about this project. I had seen no sign of new construction in the boarding school. I had heard no gossip among the students about such a grotto. I had trouble believing that a structure of the grandeur of Lourdes could somehow take root in my small village.

Later that day, I found myself standing, alongside some of my friends, all of us in our school uniforms, in front of a grotto just like those I had seen in so many reproductions as a child. Papa was standing, just as we were. There was Bernadette kneeling and the Virgin with her blue sash. I could not stop staring. The Mother Superior made a speech in which she profusely thanked Dr. Albert for his generosity. I do not believe that my father spoke. He was not someone who needed to be the center of attention.

***

All-Saints' Day was a communal holiday when we boarders enjoyed a procession that liberated us from the confines of the school walls. Wearing our uniforms, we lined up like little soldiers, two by two. An enormous colored image of a saint or the Virgin or the Patron of Deir el-Amar, Sayyidat el-Telle, or even the holy patron of the entire country, Notre Dame du Liban, was embroidered on cloth and stretched between two wooden poles.

The nuns assigned two girls to carry each image. Arms stretched in front of us, our hands would wrap themselves around one of the poles. What looked natural actually required a great deal of practice. The two girls carrying an icon had to walk together carefully and in step. If they did not, the icon would become lopsided or worse, torn from its holder.

Since the cemetery was on the opposite side of the village, the round-trip procession constituted quite an effort. What began as a daunting task swiftly became a joyous occasion. Priests and bishops in their holiday regalia led the parade, their swinging incense burners filling the air with dizzying perfume. Boys from another boarding school marched like we did, carrying their own icons. Live religious music accompanied us. The key participants, however, may well have been the Deir el-Amar natives. They stood by the side of the road, singing along with the music and clapping their hands. Neighbors, who recognized the little girls, called out their names. I always spotted Papa standing proudly and smiling encouragingly at me.

***

My First Communion took place at Les Soeurs de St. Joseph. I must have been eight or nine years old. A seamstress in the village measured me for a white dress. On this vital day in a young Catholic girl's life, I was decked out all in white: a white crown on my head, opaque white gloves on my hands, white socks and white shoes, and, of course, the white dress. After I was fully adorned, Papa had me walk around the neighborhood. As a First Communion was a very personal holiday, everyone had to see how I looked in my white outfit, just as everyone had to bestow blessings and special hugs and kisses on this rite of passage.

The day of my First Communion was terribly confusing. One of our neighbors unexpectedly gave me a present: a small shiny white prayer book and a pair of see-through white gloves. The neighbor whispered to me that this was a little something from my mother, Odette, and I was to tell no one about it. The neighbor assured me that she would inform Papa that their family was the source of the objects.

A secret? I had never had a secret to hide. My brain became a tangled web of conflicting emotions. First, I was surprised that my mother would know about my First Communion. But other feelings decided to invade my brain: amazement, disbelief, shock, panic, alarm, worry, anxiety, and most of all, fear—an enormous amount of fear. By accepting the gift, I felt I was somehow betraying Papa. My mother had been gone for so long that I could barely remember what she looked like. I was tortured by the temptation to return the entire package. But the neighbor had insisted that as far as Papa was concerned, the gifts were from that family. I loved the gloves and the shiny white book with a small colorful picture embedded in its cover. And besides, I told myself, Papa did not seem concerned about the objects. That sealed it; I decided to keep the two pieces but not be overly obvious about their existence. I discovered all-too-quickly that the see-through gloves, whose material resembled that of stockings, were doomed to a quick extinction. After wearing them a few times for masses at boarding school, the gloves began to show holes and rips, forcing me to dispose of them.

I was at once relieved and disappointed. Relieved because I no longer had to worry that their continued presence might betray their secret origin. The disappointment, however, was more deep-seated. The gloves seemed so sophisticated to my naïve eyes. I imagined that they came from a fancy store in Beirut to which I had no access. The white prayer book remains with me to this day.

***

My First Communion took place in the familiar boarding school chapel. Much to my surprise, we girls sat on the right side of the church, while, lo and behold, there were boys our age on the opposite side. I happened to be sitting at the end of the pew closest to the aisle. This provided me with a view of both the male and the female students moving up the central aisle to the altar.

As I watched the parade of boys and girls, I suddenly realized that the boys' bodies were different from those of the girls. The boys walked with their legs moving all the way up to their behinds. The girls, on the other hand, with their modest white dresses down to their calves, showed only a movement below the calves. I was convinced that the bodies of boys were some kind of aberration. After all, did not all the priests wear long robes? Sure, I was aware that Papa wore pants, but he was my father, and I had never thought of him in any other terms than being Papa.

I began thinking that there really were differences between males and females. This, I suspect, was the beginning of the sexual awareness that would blossom in me soon thereafter. To express this in words is almost sinful to me. A First Communion is a momentous religious ritual on which a child should concentrate fully. I was obviously cognizant of the fact that such a transition was spiritual. Never did I imagine, however, that the experience would involve a different sort of transition.

We young girls had practiced our First Communion ritual in advance. In this way, we were able to duly march and kneel as we had been trained to do to receive the communion wafer, with our eyes closed and our mouths open. The wafers were placed directly on our tongues by the officiating bishop.

Even before my First Communion, I helped around the church when it was time to make communion wafers. A wafer had to be a perfect circle, with no damage or crack. If a wafer happened to break in the preparation for mass, it was set aside. After all the perfect wafers were ready, those of us who helped out in the process had a chance to eat the broken fragments. Some of the students never liked the special taste of communion wafers and left the broken bits to those who really appreciated them. I was one of those who never tired of the wafer taste. As the broken part dissolved in my mouth, I would be overwhelmed by an almost spiritual pleasure at its soothing presence.

Decades later, while attending masses in New York, I began to observe the communion ritual. I was shocked to see that most Americans extended their hands, palms together, and that the priests would, without hesitation, place the wafer directly in their cupped hands. Even more painful for me was seeing individuals actually chewing the wafer.

As a child growing up Catholic in Lebanon, I learned that only the priest should touch the communion wafer once it had been transmuted into the body of Christ. Therefore, you always had to receive it directly by mouth from the hand of the officiating priest. I had also been taught that one must absolutely never chew the wafer, which must be permitted to melt slowly in your mouth. The nuns had drummed into my head that the wafer, which is, after all, the body of Christ, must not be chewed, since doing so might injure that holy body, an act tantamount to sacrilege.

CHAPTER 6

In the Mountains

Papa had numerous patients who lived in the Lebanese countryside. When I was home from boarding school, I would accompany Costy and Papa on day trips to visit the sick. For these long-distance medical journeys, Papa always had a private car and driver who remained with him until the return to Deir el-Amar, sometimes late into the night. On one occasion, a drive that began at dawn eventually led to an isolated monastery far from the village in another range of Lebanese mountains. When we arrived at our destination, Papa got out of the car, with Costy and me in tow. I took a quick glance at the monastery, an enormous stone building with multiple bell towers.

The head of the monastery and other religious figures greeted us warmly; they seemed long-time friends of Dr. Albert's. On days like this, Papa carried a large black leather medical bag containing his instruments and medications. He was shepherded to a room where he could see patients. His rounds also included bed-ridden patients. While Papa went off to his work, Costy and I were handed over to a monk, who made sure we were duly entertained. My brother and I always traveled equipped with books to read and notebooks in which we could write, as well as drawing materials, including colored pencils. We could indulge our fancy however we liked.

Costy never ceased to amaze me. Even as a child, he displayed a talent for drawing. He was able to recreate on paper something he might have seen only once. I loved the rooster he drew in its full glory in brilliant colors, wings spread and beak open, as though he were screaming at us from the sheet of paper. With his special paper and colored pencils, Costy could turn even the lemon tree in our village home into a companion that I could take to boarding school. I remain convinced that my brother Constantine inherited this ability from his namesake, our uncle Constantine.

The monks in that monastery have a beloved place in my memory. I can recall their friendly faces, their brown robes with long cowls draping from the backs of their necks and a thick, white, coiled rope loosely bound their waists, its length permitting it to hang alongside the brown robe. When the monks walked, their robes audibly swished around them.

A monk offered us food and drinks. Neither Costy nor I had a watch, but we always had a rough idea of the time by looking at the sky and watching the shadows progress on the ground. At a certain point, Papa came in to check on us. We learned that we and the driver had been invited to share the evening meal in the refectory.

I will never forget that meal. We sat with the monks on a bench at a long, wooden table in a room with an incredibly high ceiling. A monk then led us all in a prayer, sealed by our crossing ourselves. The table was already overflowing with all the Lebanese appetizers I could imagine, including fried *kibbee* (ground wheat mixed with ground lamb that was then formed into ovals and stuffed with a mixture of fried ground lamb, pine nuts, and spices, including allspice). We learned that the monastery kitchen baked fresh bread daily. It was this fresh bread that we dipped into the appetizer of our choice, be it *hummus, baba ghannouj,* or *tabbouleh* (the fried *kibbee* would be eaten with our hands).

Then the main dish arrived. To say it was delicious would be an understatement. We were served something unfamiliar: eggs boiled in a yogurt sauce subtly flavored with fresh garlic fried in olive oil and dried mint. The garlic, its perfume penetrating the entire dining room, stood out by its slightly brownish edges that provided a contrast to the white yogurt sauce. The mint that had been rubbed between the palms of the hands of the chef was visible in the specks of green that lit up the complex dish.

The rice on which the main dish rested was the typical Lebanese delicacy of rice with fried vermicelli and pine nuts that Papa made quite often. The eggs bathed in yogurt sauce were cooked perfectly. Still soft on the inside, they became one with the sauce. The bread, dipped into this exquisite specialty, picked up the subtle flavors of the heavenly mixture.

Fresh fruit topped this sumptuous meal. I watched the monks and was surprised by their lack of inhibition in their hearty enjoyment of the food. Following Turkish coffee, *de rigueur* after a meal in the Middle East, we thanked the monks profusely and they, in turn, blessed us as we embarked on the return journey to Deir el-Amar. I remember nothing about the drive home. I suspect that both my brother and I were serenaded to sleep by Papa's soothing voice as he chatted with the driver.

***

Costy was the lucky one. He was able to accompany Papa on many more medical trips than I was because I was in boarding school, and he was home-schooled by a private tutor. My brother did, however, share some of his and Papa's adventures with me, recounting mountainside picnics where Papa drank beer and smoked L&M cigarettes. My brother's good fortune was not something I envied overly. I had a problem with car drives that Costy never did. Whenever Papa had a chauffeur with a Mercedes and I rode in the back seat, I became nauseated. I remember Papa asking the driver to stop the car on many an occasion. I would then get out and vomit by the side of the road.

Once, when I was in the back of a Mercedes for the long ride from Beirut to Deir el-Amar, Papa, in an effort to make me feel better, purchased fresh bananas and offered me one. A dutiful daughter, I accepted the banana and peeled it slowly. I then took a miniscule bite of fruit and held it in my mouth as long as possible, allowing the ripe fruit to dissolve. I went to this great length to distract myself from any possible onset of nausea. By some miracle, that banana not only lasted me for the entire drive, but also prevented me from becoming nauseated.

***

One of Papa's long-distance patients became legendary in my childhood. He owned a chocolate factory. Papa never came home without some kind of goodies for Costy and me, but his return from the chocolate factory was especially memorable.

Papa entered the house as Costy and I sat playing in front of Aunt Najla's room. We both jumped up to greet and kiss our father. He was unable to grab us and lift us over his head, as was his custom. I was worried that something might be wrong. But no. Papa arrived bearing a package so gigantic that I could not even begin to wrap my arms around it. It was about half my size, and I could tell Papa clearly had trouble carrying it. I still remember Papa's laugh as he explained that this was chocolate that the owner of the factory offered to the Malti family. Papa added that the owner was not only a patient but also a longtime friend. He was aware that Dr. Albert had two young children who were sure to enjoy this special treat.

I know I had trouble believing that what Papa carried with great difficulty was actually chocolate and not some kind of strange, dark stone he had found on the road home. My brother and I simply stared at the chocolate, whose perfume was already beginning to penetrate Aunt Najla's room. None of us, and that included Aunt Najla, knew quite what to do with this object.

Papa put down his heavy package, which was still surrounded by its see-through factory wrapping. Then he went to the kitchen and utilities room adjoining Aunt Najla's personal space and returned with a hammer and ice pick. Without hesitation, he proceeded to place the pick on one edge of the chocolate and hammer it until he was able to break away chunks a child's small fingers could easily hold. Then Papa encouraged all of us to help ourselves.

I grabbed some chocolate and placed it in my mouth. I let it disappear slowly, an incredibly rich milky-chocolate taste overwhelming my senses. The small piece seemed to last forever in my mouth. When Papa urged me to take more, I did. This chocolate was around the house for some time. As soon as the small chunks began disappearing, Papa would chop off some more.

To this day, I am unable to bite into chocolate but must let it slowly melt in my mouth. I also try to convince myself that my addiction to chocolate dates to this childhood experience. Now that dark chocolate has been linked to antioxidants, and all chocolate to a chemical precursor of the neurotransmitter dopamine, I need no excuse to enjoy this sinful indulgence.

***

Early one spring morning, Papa announced that he was taking me and Costy on a trip. He was not in the habit of revealing our destinations, and this time was no exception. Costy and I were as excited as always, and we ran to ready ourselves. The driver was already at the door, prepared to head out into the Lebanese countryside. This trip was extremely long. Costy and I, when we were not busy drawing (because of my nausea, I had trouble reading in a moving car), spent our time gazing at the passing scenery. It was a drive we had never taken before. We went up and down different mountainsides. We drove through kilometers of umbrella pines. We passed streams, stopping sometimes for a drink of cold mountain water.

Finally, Papa announced that we had arrived. We were on top of a mountain, with an empty and curvy road below us. The vehicle stopped on the side of a road opposite an enormous building. As we got out of the car, Papa took our hands and stood with us. Facing us was a high stone wall protecting what looked like a castle with a red roof marked by numerous angles and chimneys. We could only see the top third of the building. Gigantic trees surrounded the structure: umbrella pines, cypress, and fruit trees in bloom.

The three of us stood gazing at this unexpected view. We could hear nothing but the songs of birds. The man-made structure was isolated, almost hidden by a forest of rich greenery. I looked up at Papa and could have sworn I saw tears in his eyes. I immediately turned my eyes away, not wanting him to discover I had witnessed his emotion. Minutes passed slowly. Finally Papa spoke. His hesitant voice signaled that he was about to divulge something of great importance. This, he revealed, was the sanatorium where he had spent many years of his life as a patient with tuberculosis.

At the time, I did not grasp the enormity of this information. Even the word *tuberculosis* was a bit too complicated for my young age. I had no idea what this affliction was. And since Papa did not mention it again, nor did Aunt Najla ever speak of it, I never understood what it meant in my father's life and in that of his family. While standing in the mountains and staring at the castle-like structure, all I understood was that Papa's words, uttered with great solemnity, represented a secret he wished to share with his two young children.

Many decades later, in America, I opened a book I had carried with me from Lebanon. It was a biographical collection of prominent individuals in the Middle East. Not surprisingly, Papa's biography was included, along with a photograph. It was then that I discovered that Papa, aside from his work at the Hôpital Laënnec, had been a Research Fellow with the Rockefeller Foundation in Paris, undertaking research on tuberculosis.

But it was Thomas Mann's *The Magic Mountain* that transported me back to Papa's time in the Lebanese sanatorium. I imagined him in that "magic mountain," but in Lebanon. There were many questions I would have loved to ask my father. How many years had he spent in the sanatorium? Did he have friends there? What was his daily life like? How did his world change when he reentered the outside world? Was this illness what made him such an ardently religious man?

CHAPTER 7

Flesh and Spirit

Papa was a great cook, and one did not need to watch him very long to realize that he truly loved this part of his life. He created a baked white spaghetti I can taste now only in my imagination. The activity I never took to well was the actual slaughter of the chicken that eventually yielded one of Papa's most delicious meals. He would enter the chicken coop and choose one of the birds. I always followed him into the coop, enchanted by how calmly he picked up a chicken by its wings with one hand while shooing away the rooster with the other.

Papa would head to the veranda facing Aunt Najla's domain and prepare for the big kill. Even though the next act repulsed me, I could not pull myself away: Papa tied the legs and wings of the chicken together just in case the bird might have any illusion of escape. Then he held the chicken's head back from its body, and, with one gesture, he hacked its head off with a heavy kitchen knife. The chicken always resisted, its decapitated body jumping around, spurting blood all over the floor, its white feathers turning red in its death throes. Papa always had a container, prepared in advance, in which he collected the blood as it drained out of the animal's body—dark red and viscous. I was never able to fully watch the life liquid draining from the animal's still-warm body. I always knew the grisly procedure was complete when Umm Zahiyya began pluming the dead bird.

Meanwhile, Papa would pour the thick blood from the bowl into a small round iron frying pan and place it over a burning gas stove. This delicate process involved monitoring the blood as it changed color until it was cooked perfectly. One or two minutes too long, and Papa's delicacy would dry out and be relegated to the garbage. The cooked blood had to be eaten fresh, at least for my father. The operation at once nauseated and intrigued me: Papa grabbing the small hot frying pan by the handle with a cloth and then sliding the round, pancake-shaped, cooked blood onto a medium-sized round plate. He always offered me a bite before he ate what to him was a healthy treat. I always refused.

Instead of walking away, however, I would sit next to Papa on the ground, my back leaning against Aunt Najla's wall. I watched closely as Papa stretched

41

his legs, and plate in hand, moved the fork ever so carefully to the brownish red pancake and cut off a small piece. In between bites, my father would look at me. I can still hear his voice telling me how nourishing cooked blood was as he offered me some, and I refused yet again his excessive generosity.

What came after was by no means a disappointment, but it was certainly anticlimactic. I would partake of a little white chicken meat, but I by far preferred the delicate stuffing lovingly mixed by Papa's bare hands—an elusive combination of rice, small pieces of fried vermicelli, fresh pine nuts, spices including allspice, and other secret ingredients.

Now, decades later, I consume very little meat. I much prefer vegetables and pasta. I am not certain how much of this reluctance might be ideological. Certainly, I cannot help but think of that bleeding childhood chicken when I stare at the cooked pieces of anything that was once a living animal.

***

Aunt Najla's section of the house featured an enormous bedroom. Entering the bedroom, I would face Aunt Najla's bed. Against the wall to my right was a mattress on which slept my great aunt. I remember her terribly thin body, but what fascinated me most was that Christ appeared to this great aunt on the opposite wall, above Aunt Najla's bed, visions she described to me before she went on to join her older relatives no longer of our world.

After my great aunt died, I often slept in her bed. On such nights, Aunt Najla serenaded me to sleep with stories from, among others, the *Arabian Nights*. Her repertoire of tales was endless, and I would lie, eyes wide open, listening to her voice while I watched the thick candle flickering in its holder. I lived on Aunt Najla's stories. Her characters inhabited my brain as soon as her words landed in my eager ears: the courageous Scheherazade, her sister who accompanies her into the palace, and the disturbed ruler who robs young women of their virginity in one night in his bed, after which he kills them. My favorite stories were those of Aladdin and those with magical journeys on flying carpets. When I listened to these adventures, I placed them in our home. The males wielding swords would be made to run up and down the stairs of the multilevel Malti house. Doors that could be opened in these tales became those of the multiple bedrooms on our top floor.

Aunt Najla's voice was at once musical and emotional. She had played the piano as a young woman. Her skills at narrating Scheherazade's tales kept me awake long after she herself fell asleep. Aunt Najla's voice changed to fit a character: at times deep, at times vulnerable, sometimes hesitant, and sometimes confident. As the candle burned down, its shadows changed, merging with the shadows of the characters in my head. I do not remember ever falling asleep, but I must have, because before I knew it, I would be lying in my great aunt's bed, with Aunt Najla already up and about. My brother Costy would also be there, reminding me that it was time for us to go collect the fresh eggs from the chicken coop, heralding a delicious breakfast.

It is only as I sit writing these words decades later that I realize Aunt Najla's tales never left my brain but installed themselves comfortably in my unconscious. It is perhaps no accident that of my published works, those dealing with the *Arabian Nights* are some of my most-read pieces.

***

One late afternoon in the spring, I was walking up the steps leading from the enormous entryway to our top floor. As I was lifting my small feet one at a time up each stair, I became aware of a delicious smell emanating on my right from the lemon tree. With each breath, I made sure to inhale the intoxicating perfume.

Suddenly, I looked further to my right beyond the lemon tree. What I saw froze me in place. There, on the high wall separating our property from that of our neighbors below, was a red devil. Not just any devil, he was the embodiment of Satan, red from horns to hooves. Unlike the image of Satan I knew from church art, this emanation was actually alive. His body with legs bent at the knees was already on the top of the wall, his two arms at his sides. His long claws were also red, but the worst thing about this creature was his face. His fiery eyes bored into mine, his red mouth spilling a horrific mocking laughter.

I remember I was barefoot and wore one of my little short-sleeved dresses. I was holding something in my arms that seemed to become heavier and heavier while I stood motionless, mesmerized by Satan's voice. Suddenly, his clawed hands moved, and he raised his bent body as if he were about to jump off the wall into our house. His movement shook me out of my lethargy, and I began to run up the remaining stairs, his laughter still deafening.

The closest door on the top floor was that of Papa's bedroom. I ran into the enormous space, but Papa was not there. Tears streaming down my face, I tried to crawl as fast as I could under the bed. The darkness that might under other circumstances have frightened me was a haven that I convinced myself could protect me from that red devil. I closed my eyes and began crossing myself and reciting the rosary. I wanted to see nothing and, most of all, I wanted to chase away that horrific laughter that had bored into my ears. I was not sure how long I remained under the bed, crossing myself and praying.

All I remember is that eventually Satan's laughter came to a halt, and I felt the presence of the Virgin Mary protecting me. I managed to slide myself from under Papa's bed and somehow found the courage to go out on the *balcon*. I looked down on the wall where that cursed creature had sat. He was nowhere to be found. To this day, I can still see his mocking face, and it does not take much concentration for me to summon up his laughter. As I write of this episode, I find myself shivering in fear of that devil who was so alive during my childhood, afire with the red of the burning Hell ever-present in my Lebanese Catholic education. Whenever I have a bad experience or undergo a trauma of some sort, that devil reappears, still laughing at me, his red color and his voice possessing, decades later, the same vibrancy they had in my childhood.

CHAPTER 8

Besançon

Not long after my First Communion at Les Soeurs de St. Joseph in Deir el-Amar, Papa transferred me to Les Soeurs de Besançon in Beirut, a more exclusive school in the Lebanese capital. To make the trip to the new boarding school more enticing, Papa always asked the driver to follow a wide two-way street that led to the school. As we approached the immense grounds, whose entrance was to our left, we passed a store on our right, where Papa had the driver stop.

The first time that Papa led me by the hand toward the shop, I stopped and gazed at the glass storefront. All I remember is being overwhelmed by the colorful display of books. My father never underestimated my love for books. But this store was special. It sold French comic strips, *bandes dessinées*, a genre more prominent in French cultural life than in America. Entering the store, I felt as if I had been transported into a world of wonder, full of color and exoticism.

I had entered a new world, the world of Tintin, the hero of the Belgian comic strips by Hergé. Papa picked up an album and placed it in my small hands. I held the book as if it were a sacred relic. My eyes landed on the colorful cover. I had never seen such an object in my life. I looked up at Papa and he was smiling at me.

"Go ahead, open the album," I heard his voice saying.

"I can't," I heard myself responding.

Papa reached down and opened the album to the first page. That simple gesture turned me into a Tintin addict. An intrepid reporter who traveled the globe, from America through Africa to East Asia, Tintin was never without his constant companion, his dog, Milou. But his escapades, not devoid of humor, would not have been the same without the cast of characters in his entourage, including le Capitaine Haddock, an old alcoholic seafarer, two hapless detectives, Dupont and Dupond, and the inimitable opera diva, La Castafiore.

To this day, when I need an escape, I bury myself in one of my Tintin albums, all newly acquired over my periods of residence in America and France. Through the decades, my favorite has been *Le Temple du Soleil* (The Temple of the Sun) in which Tintin's adventures take place in Peru, and the album is full of intrigue and mystery, not to mention the exoticism of a continent I knew nothing about until recent years. I still laugh when I see the llama spitting at Captain Haddock, and I am still mesmerized by the eclipse that saves the characters from certain death. In 2009, I noticed that certain winter headgear became fashionable, hats which looked so much like the caps with long dangling braids worn by the Peruvian characters in the Hergé album that I absolutely had to have one.

***

Directly after the Tintin store, Papa would have the driver deliver us to the enormous educational complex of Les Soeurs de Besançon. A vast, well-maintained garden with tall palm trees and flower beds swept the visitor into the walled grounds of the boarding school. The Mother Superior, who knew Papa, welcomed me as a student, and I officially became a boarder. I must have been nine or ten years old.

What I loved most about this new school were the weekly outings with the nuns. Les Soeurs de Besançon had blue buses with the school name emblazoned in white. The buses would merge with the Beirut traffic, taking up the space of multiple cars. Sitting on the buses, we little girls prided ourselves on towering over the drivers and passengers who sat in normal cars that reached barely halfway up the bus. As we waved and screamed and sang, passengers or drivers might wave back at us.

These excursions lasted for the better part of a day. After a long drive into the countryside, we would all get out, accompanied by our constant guardians, the nuns. They usually left the bus first, and as each student followed, the nun standing at the door of the bus would hand her a box containing the afternoon snack. We could guess what was most likely in the box because its contents did not vary greatly from week to week.

As we sat on the grass, we opened our boxes to find crackers, a wedge of the French cheese, *La Vache qui Rit* (The Laughing Cow), fresh fruit, and pastries—a wonderful change from boarding school fare. My favorite part was the fruit, partly because it changed with the seasons: tangerines, bananas, oranges, apples, grapes, figs, and so many others. Peeling the ripe tangerines was intoxicating. I would hold the tangerine in my left hand and pierce the top of the fruit with my right thumb. Immediately, the peel would start becoming slightly moist, as if dew had settled on it, and an indescribable perfume would overwhelm me. The intoxication continued as the tangerine went on to lose all its outer skin. When I grabbed a wedge of the fruit, the spider-like white webbing still protected it. I never removed it. It was part of the complexity of the fruit as it entered my mouth, and I would hold it as long as possible before biting into it and releasing its delicate taste. I consumed the entirety of the peeled fruit, seeds and all.

Oranges received a treatment all their own. Taking the plastic knife included in our picnic basket, I would cut a small circle around the top of the orange resting in my left hand. Once I removed the orange peel from this small area, I would insert the utensil inside the orange and move it around the fruit over and over again. I could tell the knife was tearing up the inside of the orange, but the operation was not complete until the orange was fully dissected inside its peel. Then came ecstasy. Holding the open top of the orange to my mouth and surrounding it with my lips, I would squeeze the orange with both hands. I swallowed the sweet juice as long as the orange released it.

Even then, I had not yet finished with the dilapidated fruit. Grabbing its body, by now wrinkled and bereft of its rounded form, I tore it into small pieces, one at a time. The now-damaged orange rested in my picnic container, since I needed both my hands to carry the torn piece to my mouth and bite what remained of the fruit inside the skin, seeds and all. I also loved the taste of the thin cotton-like white lining of the orange skin. I continued in this way, piece by piece, until all that remained of the original fruit was its thin orange outer skin, in pieces, relegated to the snack box that would eventually find its resting place in the Beirut garbage.

Following the fruit, we could indulge in the sweets. These were always French and not Lebanese, such as, say, baklava. This oddity never struck me when I was living in the French educational system. We had sugar cookies, biscuits layered with chocolate, coconut macaroons, little chocolate bars, and whatever the chef in the boarding school kitchen decided to include on a given day.

Wearing French school uniforms, we consumed the French cookies along with the French cheese. We easily could have been young boarding-school French girls on a trip in the French countryside. But our dark skin and hair set us apart, a constant reminder that we were not—and most importantly could never be—replicas of our Western teachers and guardians.

The nuns made sure we relaxed after the meal. We would lie on the grass and admire the scenery. Unfortunately, these adventures always had to come to an end. The special bus would once again become our home, but the return to the boarding school was always less boisterous than the venture out of the school gates.

***

While I was a boarder with Les Soeurs de Saint Joseph, I had become a girl scout (*une scoute* as we called them in French). Our experience included a great deal of climbing around the surrounding mountains. I greatly enjoyed being a *scoute* because I loved walking through the lush countryside, watching the shadows of trees on the mountainside as the sun moved in the sky. If I closed my eyes and breathed in the clean mountain air tinged with the smell of pine trees, I always felt as if this was the first time I had experienced that pleasure.

Physical exercise was part of the regimen at boarding school not only in Deir el-Amar but also in Beirut. In Deir el-Amar, the town was ideally suited for that. The nuns would lead us out of the school grounds as we made our way down the hill and below street level, where the dilapidated ruins of yet another Ottoman palace still retained some stone arches. On these arches, the nuns installed thick ropes for their students to climb. No matter how hard I tried, I was completely unable to climb the rope, never mastering the skill of wrapping my legs around it and moving them up as my arms moved up the rope. I dreaded this exercise.

But I was an even bigger failure in Beirut with Les Soeurs de Besançon. Since that school was not surrounded by ruins, our physical activities took place on the expansive school grounds. On the large lawn surrounding the buildings, the nuns had installed two metal rods with heavy rope between them. The rope was about two feet off the ground. Each student was to start running from one end of the lawn toward the rope and jump over it as she approached.

No matter how hard I tried, I could never make the jump. The nun, thinking I had somehow missed the mark, always asked me to repeat the exercise. My initial shame multiplied with my repeated inability to execute this seemingly simple act. When the nuns felt sorry for me, they would ask the gardener to lower the rope—but to no avail. I was simply incapable of doing what every other boarder could do. When one of them ran and jumped, it seemed so natural, so easy. But when I tried to do the same, I could not. Many were the times I burst into tears at my multiple failures.

I was certain that Papa learned of my misadventures. To this day, I cannot help but wonder if he was aware that I was carrying the inherited muscular dystrophy known so elegantly as Charcot-Marie-Tooth disease. In my moments of jocularity and especially when well-meaning individuals ask me what is wrong with me, I tell them that my body has won the lottery of distinction by suffering from a condition for which Jean-Martin Charcot is the flag bearer. (Pierre Marie was Charcot's student, and Howard Henry Tooth was the British neurologist who isolated the condition at approximately the same time as Charcot's team).

"After all," I always say, "if I have to carry the name of an inherited neurological degenerative condition, why not choose a world-famous name?"

For those who may not have heard of Charcot, I usually add a small phrase about this nineteenth-century physician's worldwide reputation and prominence in the worlds of medicine and psychiatry. After all, did not Sigmund Freud travel to France to study with him?

If Papa knew, he never uttered a word about this. Aunt Najla, however, in a letter I read long after I left Lebanon, noted the permanent sadness that my father carried. Having been afflicted with tuberculosis was bad enough, but to be the carrier of a crippling gene that randomly chooses which offspring to latch onto? As a child, however, I simply attributed my inability to complete the boarding school exercises to my own personal shortcomings.

***

My education, begun in Deir el-Amar with one order of nuns and followed in Beirut with another, remained essentially the same; no matter what the order, the nuns were rigorous. Up at dawn and continuing throughout the day, they instructed us in different subjects: mathematics, grammar, literature, dictation, memorization, and a variety of other subjects, including art.

Art class consisted of the nun placing an object, like a classical Greek vase, on her desk and having us draw it as well as we could. I loved art class and put great effort into my drawings. Walking up and down the aisles, the nun took her time, stopping at every desk and examining a student's work. I could not understand how she never tired of marching around, making comments about our progress. She eyed the shapes we created, the colors we used, and the forms of the bodies we drew. She made suggestions about the directions our colored pencils were taking. I remember that one of my drawings garnered particular praise from the nun. The next time Papa came to visit, I showed him the drawing, and I remember his pride at my performance.

Memorization included French classics, like *Les Fables de la Fontaine*. When the nun called a student's name, she would have to rise from her desk chair and proceed to the front of the room to recite the assigned text. Woe to the girl who could not perform. One forgotten word, and the memorization was judged inadequate. The student was forced to return to her desk, while the nun called another name. All of us were at attention as our eyes followed the next victim walking slowly to the front of the room.

The net effect? Early in my teaching career, at the University of Virginia, I was appointed in a Department of French and Linguistics that functioned as a home for strange languages, including Arabic, Japanese, Chinese, and Sanskrit. Allen and I socialized extensively with the professors of French, partly because we shared a linguistic bond (at that point, Allen was completing his PhD in French history). Jefferson's university was where I really learned to drink hard liquor, especially bourbon, and where I discovered the power of my training with the nuns in Lebanon. Much to my own shock, after guzzling a bit of bourbon, I could be easily enticed into reciting a fable from La Fontaine. I loved "*La Cigale et la Fourmi*" ("The Grasshopper and the Ant") so I would run through that in my inebriated state at the speed of lightning. And, much to my amazement, I can still do it to this day. What would the nuns say? I suspect that their possible displeasure at my drunken state would be offset by their pride at having installed French culture so effectively in a little Lebanese girl who, decades later, could drunkenly wave a French flag deep in the Virginia hills in the form of a La Fontaine fable.

CHAPTER 9

Womenfolk

At one point in my childhood—I was eight or nine years old—Papa remarried. My stepmother, Hana, much younger than my father, came from the village of Ayn Zhalta, located in the Shouf Mountains, not far from Deir el-Amar. None of us in the direct family attended the wedding, nor did any of us ask ourselves at the time if the couple had escaped to a nice spot for a honeymoon.

Papa offered Hana, among other things, a set of gold bracelets as a wedding gift. Gold bracelets are a standard present for females in the Middle East. When a baby girl is born, she is adorned with a gold bracelet embedded with turquoise to avert the evil eye. In my earliest memories, I was wearing such a bracelet. For newly married women, the gold is not merely a sign of the wealth and generosity of the husband. Women in the Middle East adorn their arms with gold as a form of security. The bracelets remain with the woman, and the more of them she slips on her right arm, the more envious her friends are sure to be, and the more financially secure she is sure to feel.

Hana was tall, thin, and beautiful, and her arrival meant changes in the upper floor of the house. The first bedroom on the side of the master bedroom became Hana's. Papa had purchased a large new wardrobe made of expensive wood. I was fascinated by this new piece of furniture. I would stand in the room watching Hana open the double doors. For me, it was a mysterious object endowed with supernatural powers. My mother Odette had never had such a wardrobe. Was that why she had disappeared from her children's lives like a genie from the *Arabian Nights*—there one minute and gone the next? Could that wardrobe be the magical space that would permit Hana to stay and not evaporate into thin air?

Soon, Hana became pregnant and gave birth to a baby girl. I was overjoyed by the new addition to the Malti family that delighted even Aunt Najla. Born on Christmas Day (Noël), the baby was baptized Marie-Noëlle. We called her Mimo for short. I fell in love with Mimo immediately. She was adorable, and everyone said she looked like me. Whenever I was home from boarding school, I tried to hold her and play with her as much as I could. Costy and I had acquired a baby sister, and he was as elated as I was. Papa had bought Costy a tricycle that he rode back and forth on the *balcon*. Sometimes, he would take Mimo for a ride while I stood behind the tricycle, holding Mimo's hands as Costy moved it slowly forward. Though technically, Mimo was our half-sister, Costy and I were too young to think in such terms. To us, Mimo was our sister—a sister we never dreamed we might have.

***

When I came home from school, I was free to indulge in fun with my brother, and we were rich in toys: a top we could spin and the painted jack-like bones of animal joints that we shook in our hands and flipped as we sat cross-legged on the ground. Playtime extended to the afternoons in the master bedroom, when Papa was taking his naps. Costy and I would sit comfortably in the large bedroom alcove facing the bed, where we played with colorful marbles, making sure not to awaken Papa. If we felt adventurous, we sneaked out through the large open bedroom window and walked single file on the thin top of the enormous metal house door until we reached the roof of Aunt Najla's kingdom. Extremely vigilant, she somehow always realized when we had accomplished this forbidden feat. She would then rush out of her own room screaming at us to get down immediately, something we could do more safely by crawling down the side of the chicken coop. Aunt Najla's screaming would awaken my father, who joined his sister in admonishing us. Aunt Najla's and my father's emotional frenzy had a reason: had not their sister died by walking on a wall, much like Costy and I were doing?

My favorite person—I have trouble calling her a toy because she was so alive to me—was a homemade doll I received from my aunt, whose mother had sewn it. The first time I held her in my arms, I noticed her fragility. She was made entirely of cloth. But what I most remember about her was her face. I touched it. The paint was beginning to chip: dark-skinned, dark eyes, black hair whose remnants barely stuck to her head. She spoke family history. I would hold her, place my face against her body, and inhale her smells in a childish attempt to become one with her. When I was home from boarding school, I often slept in Aunt Najla's room, hugging the doll close to my chest.

That hand-sewn doll lived happily for years. When my uncle, his American wife, and their two youngest children stopped off to visit us in Lebanon on their way to India, they brought me a doll in a box. I looked at her first through the plastic covering that held her stiff. She wore a pink and white frilly dress and bright pink ankle-length socks that hid her feet in little white plastic shoes. She boasted pink skin, blue eyes, and blond hair.

I did not dare take her out of her plastic and cardboard home. One of my American cousins accomplished the task while smilingly pointing out to me with a hand placed on the doll's face that this American marvel could open and close her blue eyes. She was given to me to hold, and I held her, but she felt cold and aloof. When I touched her pink cheeks, it was like touching the cold plastic container in which she had crossed the ocean. When her open eyes glared at me, they reminded of the blue glass marbles that my brother and I played with. Her blond hair reminded me of the straw in the chicken coop. I could not cuddle this alien creature. I could not move her body to conform to my own. To me, compared to her Lebanese cousin, she was dead, despite her moving eyes. I knew that nothing I did could ever bring her to life. When I immigrated to America, I left both dolls to my sister, Mimo.

CHAPTER 10

The Wailing

It was Christmas night, 1958. I was twelve years old. I fell asleep excited and happy. I had celebrated the holiday with my father, Hana, Mimo, and Costy. Like all other religious festivities in the Malti family, this one took place in the downstairs salon. A Christmas tree with bright lights illuminated the room. We had attended Christmas Mass, exchanged presents, and feasted on a luscious meal. Mimo was young enough to wander around the large space, and I was old enough to pick her up, carry her around, play with her, and kiss her from time to time.

My brother and I spent the night in the salon while Papa, Hana, and Mimo retreated to the master bedroom. In the middle of the night, I was awakened by the wailing voices of women. The sounds were persistent and loud enough to penetrate the thick stone walls of our house. In a half-awake state, I somehow realized that the women were mourning the death of my father. No matter how much I concentrate, no matter how often I transport myself to that time, I still cannot explain how it was that I knew these wailing women were lamenting my father's demise.

My memory jumps, like a cinematic cut; it is now daylight, and the next image that confronts my eyes is Papa, dressed in a black suit with white shirt and black tie, lying on some kind of slab inside the entrance of the salon. He was surrounded by all his medical degrees and his published books. He was completely still and not breathing. I suddenly realized that the wailing voices were right. I gazed at Papa, and I could swear that his eyes looked directly into mine.

A sensation I could not identify installed itself in my brain. Thoughts and questions I could not digest turned my mind into a boiling stew. Why did nothing make sense? How handsome my father looked. I was certain he had shaved that morning, because his face looked flawless. I could see him tying his black tie and adjusting it to fit perfectly over his shirt. Did he choose the black suit, or did Hana help him decide what to wear? Did he descend the two flights of stairs by himself? Did he realize how silly he looked, lying still like that in the salon, feet extended to show the soles of his shoes? Surely he knew that in the Middle East, it was considered insulting to display the soles of one's shoes. Papa would never allow me to do that. Why was he doing it himself?

Soon, the salon was crowded with people. I recognized some of the faces but not others, and I did not have much time to think about what was happening. Someone led me out of the room, across the courtyard in front of the salon and the clinic, past the lemon tree, and up the stairs. Along the way, I watched as church officials began to arrive, dressed in black, their long robes moving slowly in time with their small steps. The bishop made a special entrance, his crook announcing his appearance in advance.

I was placed in Aunt Najla's bedroom, at the end of her bed, close to the door. I felt like a marionette controlled by strings. Where was Costy? I had no idea. I leaned over the high bed, my face buried in the covers and my hands surrounding my head. I was numb. At the same time, I hated myself because no tears came out of my eyes. I kept hitting my head with my hands.

"Papa, Papa," I heard myself saying, repeating the word over and over again.

Then I chastised myself: "Shame on you. What is wrong with you? Why are you not shedding any tears?"

My hands kept pounding my head in punishment, but tears still evaded me. I cannot recall what happened next. All I know is that Papa had disappeared from our lives.

My memory jumps again. This time, I was sitting in a classroom, wearing a dark navy blue school uniform. I was no longer in the familiar surroundings of the Beirut Soeurs de Besançon. I had moved to a different and completely strange boarding school run by the same order of nuns, this time in Beabdat, deep in the Lebanese mountains. I did not need to look out the classroom windows to realize that the ground was covered with snow. My winter clothing and heavy boots told me that. The nun assigned us an exercise in composition: write about our activities over the Christmas holidays. I begin to write, unaware of what my pen was scratching on the paper. Before I knew it, the nun called my name. As required, I got up from my chair and, paper in hand, stood beside my desk and began to read words I felt certain someone else must have written.

Transformed into words, my father's death suddenly became reality, and tears began to flow down my face and onto my clothing. I felt the arms of the nun help me sit at my desk, where I continued to sob.

I do not understand why I broke apart at this exact moment. Were those the tears that should have bathed my hair and face the day after Christmas, a day that now seems far away but that had occurred barely two weeks before? Why did those tears hide for so long? Once again, I felt shame, but this time it was not at my inability to cry. It was at my lack of control over my emotions, at the looks I was sure the other students directed at me for the disruption of the class that was canceled following my outbreak. It was then that I realized that Papa was gone, that he had been stolen from me and from whatever remained of the family I had left behind in Deir el-Amar.

***

Decades later, I discovered a letter Hana had written to my uncle Michel in America. In a white envelope with a black border (signifying mourning), it was written in Arabic on a French and Arabic letterhead bearing my father's name and address. Hana had taken great care to describe in detail the events of that fateful day.

Christmas Day had begun at 8:30 a.m. when we all attended Mass. From there, Hana jumped to midafternoon at exactly 3:30 p.m., when Papa began to complain of a powerful pain in his chest. This pain eventually disappeared after an hour, but Papa was still tired. At 6:30 p.m., he decided to venture out to the churches in Deir el-Amar, as was his habit on Sundays and religious holidays, to transmit the Malti family's best wishes to all the religious dignitaries. Hence, I was not surprised to read that Papa did not return home until 10:00 p.m. At 2:30 a.m., his chest pain returned, but this time in a much stronger form. Dr. Fouad Rihan was called in, but the time of his arrival was not given. After examining Papa, the physician declared that he had suffered a heart attack, and there was no hope for a cure. In less than an hour, Papa was no longer of this world. His time of death was noted by Hana as 4:00 a.m.

The suspicion of Papa's death that reached my unconscious when the women awakened me with their wailing was unfortunately correct. Only in retrospect do I realize that we children were enjoying Christmas Day while Papa was beginning to show signs of his impending death. The vision of Papa in a black suit, surrounded by his medical degrees, remains with me to this day. Costy and I were not permitted to attend either the funeral mass or the burial.

CHAPTER 11

Upheavals

My father's death abruptly transformed my life and that of my brother, but in different ways. I was moved from boarding school in Beirut to Beabdat. Costy no longer had home schooling but was shipped off to a boarding school in Sidon: one of us in the snow and the cold, and the other in the sun on the Mediterranean. Landing among the same order of nuns in which Papa had enrolled me in Beirut was of little comfort. Gone were the stops at the Tintin store in the Lebanese capital. Gone were the weekend school bus rides, replete with picnic boxes. Gone was the large, luxuriant garden of palm trees and blooming flowers. If any comfort was to be had, it was that I was no longer required to demonstrate my failures at physical exercise.

What remains of Beabdat in my mind is my musical training. I had started learning to play the piano and sing when I first entered Les Soeurs de Saint Joseph in Deir el-Amar. I continued those studies with the Beirut Soeurs de Besançon. At Beabdat I sang in a choir in Latin during Sunday Mass. Being part of a Latin choir seemed to my young self a greater accomplishment than being a fake French sailor back in Les Soeurs de Saint Joseph. Even now, when I listen to the Christmas Eve Mass broadcast from the Vatican, I find myself singing along in Latin.

***

The death of my father in December 1958 represented more than a mere change of schools. Papa's death was an erupting volcano whose lava buried part of my life and that of Costy's. Decades after our arrival in America, my brother gave me a cache of letters from Lebanon that he had held onto for years. He could not read the ones in Arabic. When I added those to the letters Aunt Najla had written to me in America and to the contents of a folder I had taken from Michel's study after his death, I came to see how our departure from our native land had been preordained.

Reading the correspondence between my Uncle Michel, my Aunt Najla, my stepmother Hana, and that of various attorneys, priests, friends of Michel's, and so on, I understood that Costy and I had won a lottery we had not entered. Our prize: a ticket to America, to Ithaca, New York, where Uncle Michel lived. Unbeknownst to us children at the time, my uncle Michel was being bombarded with letters from different parties in Lebanon—church officials, Aunt Najla, Hana, and others—warning him of a lurking danger. That danger was made up of one word: Odette, my biological mother.

All the missives claimed that this evil woman had made her way to the village immediately following my father's demise and was living in sin with a man (in the time and place, this accusation strains credulity). Her diabolical plans included visiting her children and getting custody of them. She was simply awaiting the moment to swoop down like a hawk and carry them away like innocent rabbits. Michel was urged to move as fast as possible to get Fedwa and Constantine out of the clutches of the evil Odette.

***

One day, in the Beabdat boarding school, mere weeks after my father's death, a tall, thin nun came to my classroom, whispered some words to the sister in charge, and then moved toward my desk, gently taking my hand. I can still feel the stares of the other students burning my back as we left the room. Hand in hand, we moved down a long corridor, then down another long corridor, then into the wood-paneled room where visitors are welcomed.

I did not recognize the woman awaiting my arrival. She smiled at me.

"Your mother, Odette, is here to see you." The nun's words beat on my ears as on a drum.

Odette—the mother who had vaporized into thin air when I was four years old? My last vision of her, almost eight years before, was of a woman screaming and fighting, broom in hand, with Aunt Najla. Odette stood when the nun and I entered the room. The nun still held my hand as she led me to my mother, who bore a large white box wrapped with ribbons. I was overwhelmed by the smell of coconut macaroons. Was that what was hidden in the box?

I have no memory of my mother hugging me, but I cannot believe she did not. My mother was a tall, beautiful, young woman elegantly dressed in black. The black of mourning was standard in the Middle East. She could not have been mourning the death of my father, since they were no longer together. Was she mourning the loss of another spouse?

My hand was still in that of the nun who led me to a baby grand piano to the left of the room entrance, next to the shiny wooden bookshelves that rose from floor to ceiling. The nun released my hand, and I sat on the bench. My hands now free, I was ordered to perform for my mother. I dutifully played a piece of classical music I had been taught. I concentrated on the movement of my fingers in a mad effort to distract myself from the odor of coconut macaroons wafting toward me from the box next to my mother.

After completing the piano piece, I moved toward my mother, whose hand beckoned me to sit. She opened the box. Ah! It was, as I suspected, full of coconut macaroons. What my memory retains was the smell and the taste. Odette offered me the box, and I refused, as I was required to do by Middle Eastern rules of politeness. I finally took one macaroon. Ever so slightly brown on the top as it should be, the macaroon rested in my right hand while I admired it. I could tell it came from an expensive bakery in Beirut because every bite was a complex mix of soft dough with a slight crunch and generous shreds of fresh coconut. My mother watched me as I finished one. She quickly encouraged me to take another. I refused, as I should. Once again, we played that familiar game, and only then did I succumb. I convinced myself that the delicacies were at least keeping my hands and mouth busy, distracting me as my mother talked.

She spoke first. After the usual niceties, she got to the point.

"I know that your father's family is trying to take you away from me and send you and Constantine to America. Did you know that?"

I answered by nodding my head yes, mouth full of the Beirut delicacy.

"Do you want to go to America?"

I shrugged my shoulders, since I knew it was impolite to speak with food in your mouth.

"Have they said anything to you about it?" As if I were a puppet pulled by invisible strings, my head nodded a "Yes."

"Have they asked you if you want to go?" This time, I shook my head "no."

"When they ask you if you want to go to America, you should say no."

I was chewing slowly, concentrating on the complicated flavors of the macaroon in the hope they would block my mother's voice.

"You must do that."

I mumbled something that expressed my powerlessness.

"I know that there are important people involved in this. Are you afraid of them?"

"Yes."

"You shouldn't be, my daughter."

Odette put her arms around me and hugged me. I sensed that she was trying to protect me.

"You do know that I love you and Constantine very much, don't you?"

"Yes," I answered in an unsure voice. I really did not understand how she could love me and Costy, since she had vanished from our lives without so much as a goodbye.

"Do you think you could tell those who ask you if you want to go to America that you would rather stay in Lebanon?"

I did not know what to say, so I did not reply.

This conversation was making me extremely uncomfortable. My legs were moving back and forth under the bench, and I felt my body shrinking, as if it were disappearing. My mother seemed oblivious to my unease. Her final words to me, delivered in her fluent French, were permanently engraved on my brain: "*Si on veut on peut*" (If one wants, one can).

If I had known then what I know now, I would have responded, "Not always." I did not really want to go to America, but I was thirteen years old, my brother was ten, and our destinies were not ours to choose.

My mother was relentless: at times cajoling, at times begging, and at times pressuring. I tried to concentrate on the macaroons sitting safely in their box. Their powerful scent had already infused the room. My discomfort during the entire visit was so powerful, I was sure it would shatter me into pieces. With great hesitation, I muttered that no one was asking my opinion in this matter. Only later in life did I learn that my uncle in America had been working to have my brother and me shipped off to his country of adoption, a land he called "Paradise on earth." Had I said a word, it would have remained unheard among the voices of church officials, family members, and attorneys. Odette's journey had been in vain, save, of course, for the macaroons.

The encounter with my mother must have occurred sometime in the winter, shortly after Papa's death. The woolen dark navy school uniform I wore that day tells me that. How did the visit end? My memory is blank. What I remember of Beabdat must have melted with the snow that covered the surrounding mountains, a winter that seems in my memory to have lasted the entire time I was there. Odette vanished, and I do not remember saying goodbye to her. I do remember being overwhelmed with guilt that I had somehow disappointed her. It was the first time I had seen my mother since her disappearance from our lives eight years before. I would not see her again for another twenty years.

***

My stay with Les Soeurs de Besançon in Beabdat remains a blank but for the snow, my musical studies, the tears I shed in the classroom over the essay about my father's death, and my mother's visit with the coconut macaroons. I spent, after all, several months in Beabdat. The only reason the music room stands out in my memory is because it was directly across from the visitors' room, and I glanced at it, admiring its steps, as the nun led me by the hand to see Odette. But if I concentrate too long on the steps, even the music room begins to dissolve in my memory. Was that space actually the small chapel where masses were held? If I dig deep enough in my memory, though, I am able to unearth one additional image: the side of the school building with its overflowing garbage cans. All my attempts to replace this unsightly vision with something more edifying are failures. What I know for certain is that I completed my studies at Beabdat at the end of the term and found myself back in my village of Deir el-Amar. Did Hana, my stepmother, accompany me back to the family home? A blank page is all I see, and I am unable to fill it in, even when I attempt to do so with an imaginary reality.

***

The house in Deir el-Amar to which I returned was not the house from which I had departed when I left for Beabdat. Though I knew that Papa was no longer of this world, I nevertheless expected him to walk through the large entrance of our home at any moment. I had convinced myself that my time in Beabdat was an anomaly. I expected Papa to greet me as I entered the house, hugging me and lifting me in the air as he always did. I expected him to be in his clinic treating the ill, with patients waiting their turn on the bench outside. I could swear I heard their chatter as I headed down the stairs to the lowest level of the house. Soon, I realized that a new stillness pervaded the house. Sure, I could hear isolated voices, those of Aunt Najla, Hana, Mimo, Umm Zahiyya, and Costy. But the indescribable energy that had always infused our enormous stone abode was now gone. I felt like a disembodied ghost, floating in an unfamiliar place. Whatever had once held my life together had now utterly disappeared.

CHAPTER 12

Paradise on Earth

That infamous folder I recovered after Michel's death, and which I renamed the "adoption folder," proved a veritable treasure. My uncle Michel apparently kept every scrap of paper relating to his family back in the old country. Michel had exchanged correspondence with a Dr. Edward Mikol, General Director of Tuberculosis Hospitals for the State of New York Department of Health, in October 1957 in what turned out to be a futile attempt to bring my father and the extended family to America. I also learned that Papa had received all his medical degrees from Beirut and the Faculty of Medicine in Paris by 1930, when he was twenty-five. His specialty was tuberculosis and pulmonary medicine. When I look back at his life and his late marriage to Odette, I draw the unpleasant conclusion that he most likely contracted tuberculosis from one of his unfortunate patients. How long did he spend in that sanatorium in the Lebanese mountains that he was so intent on showing to Costy and me?

Michel's plans to have his brother and the entire family become Americans having come to naught, he proceeded, following Papa's demise, to attempt to import the remainder of his Lebanese relatives to America. To that end, Aunt Najla, in her most meticulous English handwriting, carefully drafted a chart listing the five family members (including Costy and me) along with pertinent information, like dates of birth. The heavy blue sheet of paper, carefully cut down to the part containing the vital information, remains in my memory. Decades later, in my mind's eye, I can still see Aunt Najla sitting in her room, carefully composing the chart.

Correspondence flowed like ocean currents from the Levant to America. The numerous complicated American immigration documents reveal Michel's assiduous labor, as letters from members of Congress, including the Majority Leader of the Senate at the time, Lyndon B. Johnson, were submerged under the enormous paperwork. How strange to discover that the collection of Lebanese Maltis ("Najla," "Hanna," "Fadwa," "Constantin," and "Marie," as our names are spelled in House Bill H.R. 6085 and in Senate Bill S. 1890) had become part of the American legislative process.

In the Senate bill, preserved in that folder, all of us were "considered to be nonquota immigrants." Why was this? Because early on in the process, a communication from the Department of State addressed to Senator Kenneth Keating of New York makes it clear that:

> The quota for Lebanon, to which I assume they are chargeable for immigration purposes, has been heavily oversubscribed for some time. Consequently, persons recently registered under that quota must anticipate a protracted delay of indefinite duration before nonpreference numbers from that quota will become available for their use.

We were members of an enormous throng of Lebanese citizens who were looking for ways to improve their lives.

All this transpired while Costy and I were separately plunked in our respective boarding schools. "Moreover," Michel writes to his attorney in Ithaca, "it is essential, for the sake of the three children, that they have somebody who could act as a father in bringing them up to be useful citizens." In a letter addressed to his longtime friend, Mustafa Khalidy, a physician and member of the well-known Khalidy family, Michel bares his soul. He wonders about the different possibilities facing him.

> Again, suppose that I meet with failure in the matter of getting the two older children into the States. How would these children be cared for from a disciplinary point of view? I suppose that they could be sent to boarding school during nine months, but how about the other three months of the year? Fadwa would not be too much of [sic] trouble. But Constantin needs the firm hand of a man to keep him under control.

"[T]he firm hand of a man." That no one understood the implications of such an image strikes me only now as I write these words. It was after we arrived in America that both Costy and I experienced that "firm hand of a man." Papa did not believe in corporal punishment. At times, I can only wonder how these two males, so different in their outlook on family matters, were born of the same seed.

Michel always had the right answer. In the same letter to his friend, he makes it clear that:

As to asking Fadwa [sic] and Constantin [sic] whether they would like to emigrate, I feel that we should endeavor to do what is best for them regardless of their views. I would not mind knowing these views but can not [sic] promise to carry out their wishes if they conflict with my ideas of what serves their best interests. If their views are negative, I am sure that Najla could change them by talking to the children. I hope you agree with my attitude on this matter.

Having never met Mustafa Khalidy, I can only wonder what this physician's reaction would have been to Michel's missive. Why do I wonder? Because directly following this paragraph comes this request:

When you write again, please have this letter in front of you and try to comment on every point I have raised. I have an open mind and I am willing to listen to ideas and suggestions especially when they come from a friend whom I trust.

My uncle Michel was not one to write such a letter on the spur of the moment. Instead, he always drafted a longhand copy that he then consigned to the typewriter. He and Mustafa had been longtime friends and wrote endlessly to one another about political issues dear to their hearts, like the Palestinian situation.

Encountering these documents, so long ignored on the bottom of a shelf in my home library, evokes a strange mixture of sensations in me. It is as if I were back in our salon in Deir el-Amar, listening to the women wailing and somehow knowing the sound signals my father's death. The image of my father in his dark suit lying in the salon surrounded by all his medical degrees and books intrudes on my consciousness. I have spent more years on earth than my own father, who died at age fifty-five, and I cannot comprehend how I have lived longer than he did. I feel strangely disembodied when I read my name in that old American official correspondence. There I was, pursuing my studies in Beabdat, completely unaware that there was a Fedwa who existed in the same universe as Lyndon B. Johnson. That entity named Fedwa (or Fadwa as she is spelled in the documents of that time) is completely unfamiliar to me. At times, even her gender changes, as some documents refer to her and Costy as Michel's "nephews."

***

As late as April 1959, four months after my father's death, it appeared that the entire Malti clan was still slated to undertake the voyage to America, even though as early as February 10, 1959, Aunt Najla had written her brother Michel concerning me and my brother. She tells him "to take them as soon as possible because now the bishop permitted their mother to see them. She goes there often and is trying to change their minds." The bishop in question was the leading official of the Melkite Catholic Church to which our family belonged.

Much more significant, however, Aunt Najla clearly states she did not wish to go to America because she could not travel and she and Hana were living peacefully. Michel's quest ultimately led exactly to what Aunt Najla had written in February. She, Hana, and Mimo would remain in Lebanon while my brother and I left our native country for America. Years later, I heard another explanation for this decision: the US government refused Aunt Najla a visa because of her poor health, and Hana decided to stay behind with her and Mimo. Finally, my uncle had to adopt Costy and me because the only other option, student visas, would have required us to return to Lebanon after our studies.

My brother and I left our boarding schools and arrived home in Deir el-Amar, unaware of the drama that had been playing for months to an avid audience in the village. There was the evil Odette who, according to the Archbishop of the Melkite-Catholic Church and a close friend of the Malti family, was married and wished to gain custody of her two children. From Aunt Najla and Hana came the more traditional narrative: Odette was living with a man to whom she was not married. Facing down all this evil was an angel of salvation, the Archangel Michael—that is, my uncle Michel from America. It seemed that everyone in the village, with the exception of the two individuals in question, knew that Fedwa and Constantine were about to be shipped off to America.

CHAPTER 13

Preparing the Emigrants

I did not fully understand when I left Beabdat and Les Soeurs de Besançon that I was making a final departure—that this would be our last summer in Lebanon. Constantine and I were to leave for the United States in August 1959, in time to begin the new school year in America.

A newly-purchased white radio perched high on a shelf greeted me as I entered Aunt Najla's room, transforming the space into a social center for older neighborhood women who sat, legs crossed in the Middle Eastern manner, on the floor of the room, listening to the radio. (Aunt Najla received a weekly written guide advising listeners of available programs.) I could not be certain whether the women were digesting the sounds flying from that strange machine. They exchanged gossip, laughed out loud, drank Turkish coffee prepared by Umm Zahiyya, and indulged in fresh pastry prepared for the occasion. Whenever I entered the room, they would ululate and clap their hands. At first, their actions took me aback. Later, I understood the reason for this joyous behavior.

They were excited about the two Malti children's departure to America. There was no television in the village, but these women knew of its existence in the far-away land to which Costy and I were headed. I cannot possibly count the number of times they asked me to please get on the television in that distant place and speak to them. Of course, I was just as ignorant of television as they were and always agreed to their requests. Whenever I sit in a television studio in the United States, memories of Aunt Najla and her friends in Deir el-Amar beseeching me to speak to them through the magical machine overtake me, and I realize again how naïve we all were in our insular mountain environment.

***

That last summer in Lebanon was so overwhelming that I have trouble remembering it. That last summer in Lebanon became isolated episodes so intense they overwhelm and destroy any other events in their path. That last summer in Lebanon, despite or perhaps because of its intensity, flew by as quickly as the swiftest bird.

Hana took me to the St. Elias Church to obtain the first of many blessings I would receive for the upcoming trip to the United States. I sat on the padded bench across from the desk behind which the Bishop made himself comfortable. He and Hana exchanged small talk as his wife offered his guests hot drinks and pastry. My legs dangled, unable to reach the floor below. I began to move them back and forth, one forward, one back, then one forward, one back—over and over.

The stern voice of the religious authority cut through my reverie: "Fedwa," he began. "You must not do that. It is very bad. Americans never do things like that, and you have to learn how to behave in America." I said nothing but stopped moving my legs. I could not help but wonder about this new country to which we were being shipped.

Back home, I was fed other tales about America. Since Costy and I were the only ones about to enter my uncle Michel's "Paradise on earth," all responsibilities for Costy's safety fell on me.

"Your brother is younger than you. You must take care of him and keep him safe," Aunt Najla told me one day. But telling me once was not enough. She repeated this mantra to me daily, often more than once a day. Then one afternoon, Aunt Najla and her friends began relating stories about what happens to children in America. If a youngster went out alone, I learned, he or she would be kidnapped and sold to unspecified buyers. Some evildoers even stole children to kill them.

One tale made such an impression on me that I remember it to this day. Africans, I learned, were in the habit of kidnapping young children in public places like airports or empty streets, then taking them to hidden locations where they would proceed to cut their bellies open and stuff their abdomens with drugs. This way, drug dealers entering a country were safe, since they would be carrying a child. The storytellers emphasized that somehow the stolen child remained alive during the operation and while transporting the drugs. The image of my brother in such a state frightened me to the point of tears every time I heard the story.

Africans? These women made them seem huge and terrifying. I was not sure who these so-called Africans were. I had learned about Africans from the nuns, but nothing that cast them in a bad light. Papa had medical pamphlets in his consultation room with pictures of African nuns, alongside European nuns, ministering to the ill in Madagascar and other French colonies.

All the women at these gatherings felt the need to elaborate on the moral of these cautionary tales, lest I not understand them. I must watch Constantine constantly. I should not let him move anywhere without holding his hand. I was responsible for my brother's safety and wellbeing. This literally put the fear of God into me. If anything bad were to happen to my brother, I would be to blame. Guilt, instilled in me as a younger child by the nuns, was now moving into higher gear.

***

As summer progressed, our August departure for America loomed on the horizon like a giant storm. We began receiving correspondence from some of Michel's grown children. I was certain these missives were meant as gestures of welcome from America. But to us back in the village, the individuals penning these letters were exotic strangers whose existence in a far-off land had only become known to us after Papa's death.

My uncle Michel's oldest daughter, a graduate of Cornell University, wrote to us. Aunt Najla opened the letter, hand-written in English. Fortunately, she was able to decipher the writing scribbled on two pages in blue ink from a fountain pen. Costy and I sat cross-legged on the stone courtyard floor next to Aunt Najla, her bedroom outside wall supporting her back. Each of us children leaned on one of Aunt Najla's legs as she slowly read and translated the contents of the letter. At the time, these letters did not make much sense to any of us, but one word stood out in Aunt Najla's studious deciphering: Dad. Dad? Aunt Najla had no idea what this word meant and, of course, neither did us children.

When I look at the blotchy letter half a century later, I cannot help but muse on its peculiarities. There are ink smudges throughout the text, indicating that the fountain pen rested more than it should have on certain letters. The right margins vary; in some the words hug the end of the page, and in others the lines take up only one third of the available space. Even more provocative is what we learned about the family: "We, as a family, enjoy working, playing, talking, and reading together." The letter "f" of family shows signs of having had the pen dwell too long on it. The word *together* lies at a steep angle, hanging between three lines, as if it had been inserted as an afterthought.

We learned from the letter that the married couple and their three children lived in Williamstown, Massachusetts.

Williamstown is in northwestern Massachusetts,

state   state

near the New York ^ and Vermont ^ borders. Perhaps you can find it on
a map.

In the village, all these strange names jumbled together in my mind. And
then there were two of their children: "David and Faith spend most of every
day playing together, pretending house and store and lots of other things."
In the stone courtyard, sitting next to Aunt Najla, we found all of this utterly
incomprehensible.

Yet another missive in English arrived from another of Michel's grown children,
this time from his fourth daughter. A., also a graduate of Cornell University, had
married a farmer. Costy and I learned about this family, once again from Aunt
Najla's translation. The daughter explained that she fed the "calfs" [sic], swept the
barn, and turned the cows out to pasture. We were promised a ride on a horse
upon our arrival at the farm. Costy received an additional treat: he "may ride on
the big tractors." Tractors? Neither Costy nor I had any idea what these were. I
wondered why only Costy could ride the "big tractors" and not me.

This particular daughter was much more industrious than her older sister.
Wishing to begin the education of her two young Lebanese relatives, she writes:

I have some words below here that I would like Constantine to try
and read.

1. cow   2. horse
3. dog   4. baby
        5. farm

Let me know if he could [sic] read them. I'm sure Fedwa could.

I have no memory of Aunt Najla asking either Constantine or me to read those
unfamiliar words. Did she translate them for the two of us? I cannot be certain. I
felt confused by this distant and alien universe we were about to enter. Nor could
I comprehend the need for one of Michel's daughters to test our English reading
skills. To this day I still search my brain for how I might have pronounced the
word *cow* and cannot imagine generating the correct pronunciation.

Many were the nights during that last summer in Lebanon when I cried myself to sleep. I was certain I had shed all the tears I could over Papa's untimely death, but I quickly learned that the body holds oceans of tears, whose waves crash at unexpected times, drowning the mind. Aunt Najla, however, always felt encouraged and optimistic when we received letters from our American relatives. At times, I wonder if these missives assuaged her guilt at shipping my brother and me to an unknown land.

***

We spent much of that summer in Lebanon preparing to embark on our journey to a strange world with whose language, food, and customs we were not familiar. Hana was excellent at organizing, and she arranged all the tasks we had to complete before our departure. Most important among these realms we were about to pass through was the Lebanese government bureaucracy. Neither Costy nor I had a national identification card.

Hana walked me and Costy to the government office in Deir el-Amar in charge of identity cards. The office was located in the front section of the famous Ottoman prison that I passed every time I walked home from the boarding school of Les Soeurs de St. Joseph. The building had always been an object of fascination, and setting foot in it was at once thrilling and frightening. There were forms to complete and police filling the room. Fortunately, Hana was holding my hand. I tried to convince myself to be brave.

Both Costy and I needed photographs for these documents. When I look at my card, what stares back at me is an angry face I barely recognize as my own. My hair had been cut short. No smile adorned my rebellious face. I was wearing my dark school uniform, which tells me that the mountains must have been cold when I posed. My first Lebanese passport shows me with longer hair and a summer dress. My face, however, still looks at me with an accusatory eye and no smile.

***

Our greatest adventures prior to departing our native land that summer were the multiple trips to Beirut. Hana had enlisted her brother to accompany her, Costy, and me. I did not understand at the time the importance of having a male relative as a companion. Now I know it would have been unseemly for a single woman, even with two children in tow, to travel alone to the big city. After my father's death, Hana, like all Middle Eastern widows, wore black and dutifully tucked her hair into a bun at the back of her head, covering it with a black scarf when she left the house. Mimo, still a baby, did not accompany us on these day-long journeys, remaining at home with Aunt Najla and Umm Zahiyya.

The main purpose of our trips to the Lebanese capital was shopping, something unfamiliar to both Costy and me. I suspect there was a great deal of pride at stake on this buying spree. After all, Costy and Fedwa were off to America, and no one in the family, or for that matter in the entire village, wanted Americans to think that we Lebanese were backward or inferior. We meandered from shop to shop, acquiring new clothing for Costy and me. Costy's outfits were those of a well-dressed French boy: matching shorts and jackets. These new suits only added to my brother's natural good looks—good looks he has conserved to this day. The largest objects we purchased were two enormous suitcases, among the biggest I have ever seen. The suitcases were light blue and had dark blue handles and leather straps.

On one of these shopping trips, Hana organized a surprise for us. We were to go on a boat ride on the Mediterranean. It was a beautiful, sunny summer day in Beirut, and neither Costy nor I had ever been on the sea. Once we were all on the boat and floating majestically on the clear blue water, I was overwhelmed by emotion. As I breathed in the exotic smell of the sea, I could only stare around me in a daze. Voices and noises coming from our boat as well as other boats filled my ears. I was unable to utter a word. I felt insignificant in the presence of the majestic body of water that stretched to the horizon.

I was sure that the enormous Pigeon Rock, one of Beirut's landmarks, visible in the distance, was beckoning to me, attempting to seduce me into sailing toward its imposing mass. The calm water rocked me, as a mother rocks her child in her arms. I closed my eyes and inhaled the sea air. Suddenly, my mind began exploding, not only with the Bible stories the nuns had taught us, but also with tales from the *Arabian Nights* that Aunt Najla had related when I slept in her bedroom—the magical lamp that, when rubbed, gives birth to a genie on the seashore, Sinbad the sailor, mermaids, and Jonah and the whale. Adding to these stories were the medical booklets in Papa's clinic that featured nuns working in a hospital on the island of Madagascar, pictures in whose background stretched deep ocean water. Floating on the Mediterranean Sea that day allowed my imagination to run free. I began to comprehend the mythical qualities of these bodies of water and their attraction for storytellers. At the same time, being surrounded by the blue water as far as my eyes could see made it difficult for me to conceive of a world beyond that water.

***

When we returned to Deir el-Amar, I was in for more surprises. Aunt Najla was about to reveal secrets she had kept for decades. One day, when Hana was not at home, Aunt Najla approached me when I was in the front courtyard sitting on the cement bench and talking to my friend, Marie. My aunt wanted me to come with her. Marie, taking the hint, left. Aunt Najla took me by the hand and led me to the room adjoining her bedroom. She then turned and faced her tall, locked metal closet, and I found myself next to her. Aunt Najla whispered to me that this little escapade had to remain a secret.

"Do you understand, Fedwa? This is very important," she asked me in a whisper.

"Yes, I do," I found myself replying.

In truth, however, I did not understand at all. But I realized that if I asked too many questions, I would never be privy to what Aunt Najla was about to reveal.

Aunt Najla took a key out of her pocket and proceeded to unlock the metal closet, never before open to my gaze. She then pulled the key from its lock and placed it securely back in her pocket. As I watched, she first opened one of the doors, and then its partner. The sound of creaking metal struck my ears, making me aware that both Aunt Najla and I were in an eerily silent and enclosed space.

The two gray doors stood at attention like guards protecting the entrance to a royal treasure room. However, I found not glittering jewels but gray metallic shelves—at least six of them, as I remember. Adding to the mystery, I could see only the edges of the top shelves. I looked at Aunt Najla, but her eyes appeared mesmerized by the contents of the closet. My aunt then extended her right arm toward one of the higher shelves, obscuring what she now held in her hand.

She turned and faced me, showing me a small glass bottle in the shape of a bulldog with a painted red ribbon around its neck. The dog's little features were etched in the glass and then highlighted with thin black lines that showed signs of wear. My eyes must have given away my fascination with this unusual object. How did I know this? Because Aunt Najla laughed in an uncharacteristic, almost giggly way.

"Fedwa," she turned to me with a full smile, "do you know what this is?" I had no idea and said so.

"This small bottle," I heard her saying, "held perfume."

Perfume? I was quite confused, and this confusion turned to embarrassment when I noticed Aunt Najla staring at me.

"Yes, my little Fedwa," she continued, giggling. "This little glass dog was a perfume bottle that someone gave me as a present when I was young."

I was speechless. Perfume and Aunt Najla were not a pairing my brain could easily entertain. Questions filled my head. Who had given Aunt Najla the perfume? A secret admirer? A not-so-secret admirer? She had mentioned her youth, but I had never thought of Aunt Najla as other than the individual I had known since I was a child: overweight, gray hair in a bun, wearing homemade clothing, and having difficulty walking.

Now I was confronted by an altogether different image of my aunt. I knew she had been a school teacher. But at some point in her life as a young woman, she had decided to dedicate herself to my father, her brother. When did this change occur? I could not help but wonder if it was related to Papa's tuberculosis and his stay of many years at that sanatorium in the Lebanese mountains.

I was tantalized by the possibility that Aunt Najla had had an amorous life. She had never uttered a word about it, and yet she had kept this empty dog bottle, taking care to stash it in the metal cabinet that kept it safe from prying eyes. Why had she not disposed of the empty bottle that no longer even hinted at the perfume it once held? How often did she open the enormous metal closet and hold the tiny bottle in her hand?

Then unexpectedly, Aunt Najla, perfume dog bottle in hand, broke the silence. "My beloved Fedwa," she began, "I want you to take this bottle as a gift from me." I was flabbergasted.

"I can't, Aunt Najla," I said.

"Why not?" she replied.

"I just can't," I continued.

My response had nothing to do with the Middle Eastern politeness ritual in which you must refuse at first what you are offered. I was careful to add, "because this is something that belongs to you, and you have kept it for many years."

"That's true," she said. "But I want you to have this bottle with you in America."

"Why?"

"Because you will come to understand, Fedwa, that objects like this little glass dog are only important because they remind you of something, of someone.

When you are very distant from your Aunt Najla, you will see this bottle, and when you touch it, you will think of me and my love for you."

As I began to cry, Aunt Najla hugged me, and when her own tears moistened my hair, I realized how much she wanted me to have the glass dog.

"Oh, Aunt Najla, thank you, thank you, thank you. I will cherish this little dog as if he were a part of me."

I never imagined that Aunt Najla might have experienced an existence other than spinsterhood. That there was a time when she was young and beautiful, a time when she might have walked normally without those "upside-down champagne bottle legs," as the medical profession designates the ravages of the Charcot-Marie-Tooth form of muscular dystrophy. Now that I myself display those "upside-down champagne bottle" legs, I think often of Aunt Najla and of my childhood innocence about life.

After giving me the little glass bottle, Aunt Najla locked up the metal closet and its objects that held meaning for her alone. As I heard the key turn in the lock, I felt great disappointment. I was desperate to know what other secrets that closet might be hiding.

Aunt Najla must have read that disappointment in my face. "Don't worry, my beloved Fedwa," I heard her say as she took my hand and guided me back into her bedroom, "you and I will revisit my secret place very soon."

Sure enough, a few days later when the house was once again empty, Aunt Najla took me again into her private world. On this second visit, Aunt Najla pulled out a gold watch fob that had belonged to my grandfather, who she had told me many times had been an Ottoman medical officer who died of typhus acquired while tending to sick soldiers during World War I. She had retained the watch fob embedded with precious stones in her secret closet. Now she was offering me this extraordinary piece of family history. The gold ball shone in the sunlight, while its glittering jewels cast a rainbow of color on the wall of the crowded room. I held that piece of jewelry in my hand as Aunt Najla explained its importance. But I was much too young to appreciate what she was transmitting to me. What I could appreciate was the beauty of the shining sphere as it played with the sun.

Now a large picture of my grandfather in his Ottoman military uniform hangs in my library, a picture Costy took from our uncle's home in Florida. My brother has never revealed to me how he acquired the enormous portrait, but he did tell me that he received a call one day from one of Michel's grown children asking for it.

"You know that I have a picture of Grandma hanging in our house," she apparently began her little speech. "Could you send me the picture of Grandpa that you have? I think it would be wonderful to hang the picture of Grandpa next to the picture of Grandma, don't you? That way they can still be together."

One of the qualities that makes my brother so wonderful is that no one can intimidate him, even though his life since our arrival in America has been brutal, both emotionally and physically. His response to Michel's daughter made me laugh.

"You're absolutely right," he answered her. "Having pictures of Grandma and Grandpa Malti together would be wonderful. So why don't you send me Grandma's picture so that I can hang it next to Grandpa's?" According to my brother, Michel's daughter did not respond, but she never again asked Costy for that portrait. Whenever I walk into my home office and look at my Grandpa in his military uniform returning my stare, I imagine him dressed in a civilian suit, wearing that gold fob so generously given to me by Aunt Najla.

***

Time came to have no existence for me during those last months in Lebanon. Costy and I were the talk of the village. After all, how many people from Deir-el-Amar had been chosen to depart for America?

Aunt Najla, confined to the house, was quite pleased when Costy and I returned from Beirut with Hana and her brother, new clothing and two enormous suitcases in tow. The large bags inspired my aunt to indulge herself. For the first time, I had a chance to see some of the goodies she had hoarded in the back of her bedroom. While Costy played with his friends, Aunt Najla invited me to sit in her room as she unearthed treasures that had been buried for decades. I can still see myself watching her take one piece of cloth after another, first holding up the embroidered material for me to admire, then carefully spreading the pieces on my lap, where she encouraged me to feel them. As I did so, she explained which women family members had spent hours toiling over the colorful embroidery. From large thick cotton and silk tablecloths and napkins to silk dresses and men's shirts, from names of former generations of Malti women down to herself, Aunt Najla wove her memories through each piece. The dining-room linen, bedroom sheets, and sofa covers were household gifts for Michel and his family. What remained was clothing intended for Costy and me.

Aunt Najla isolated a dress that she was careful to offer me. Made of reddish-orange silk, the long dress had belonged to the youthful Aunt Najla. She elaborated extensively on this dress that she held up to her enormous body and that she could no longer wear. She had exquisitely embroidered it with flowers and birds in bright colors from red to green. As Aunt Najla held up the dress for my admiration, I noticed that it had an enormous rip across the top. I said nothing, not wishing to break the fairytale atmosphere in which my aunt was floating. She said nothing about the tear. I wondered at the time whether she even saw it. My aunt then divided material between the two cases, one of which would be registered in my name and the other in Costy's. With Costy's and my help, Hana and Aunt Najla packed the two large suitcases while Costy and I had each somehow earned an over-the-shoulder tote from KLM, the airline that would fly us from Lebanon to America.

Aunt Najla's parting words still reverberate in my ears. "Take care of your brother," she enjoined yet again. "He is younger than you are, and his health is more fragile."

On the day of departure, the whole family crowded into a car for the drive from Deir el-Amar to the Beirut airport. What sticks in my mind is sitting in the back of the car, directly behind the driver. I glued my face to the window as the car left the village and began the curvy descent to Beirut. I sang over and over to myself the French version of Auld Lang Syne:

"Ce n'est qu'un au-revoir, mes frères,
ce n'est qu'un au revoir ...

At times, I substituted *mes soeurs* (my sisters) for *mes frères* (my brothers). Tears flooded my eyes as I stared at the Shouf Mountains speeding by. My memory is of being completely alone, yet Costy, Hana, and Mimo must have been in the car with me. Was Aunt Najla there as well? I cannot say for sure. I am certain we hugged and kissed each other goodbye and promised to stay in touch. My brother and I walked to the airplane together.

PART II

Michel

CHAPTER 14

Hand-Off

Constantine and I were seated in the back row of the plane, with my brother near the window and me on the aisle. The flight attendant realized that I could speak French, so there was no need for an Arabic-speaking attendant. We both sat quietly, looking out the small airplane window at the Beirut airport as other passengers walked toward the plane, climbing the stairs to enter what to me was an enormous machine swallowing all of us in its long oval belly. I could not see family members easily behind the airport glass. What I could distinguish were hands waving and blowing kisses. Did those hands belong to our family? I would like to think so.

Costy and I sat, neither of us uttering a word—staring out the small window. We were both crying, and the flight attendant was attempting to calm our fears. As the plane moved down the runway, the voice of the captain serenaded us with words neither of us understood. I simply stared out the window, and as we reached our altitude, I was overcome with awe. To my young mind, we were floating on the very clouds I would gaze at in the sky from our house in the village. It seemed almost miraculous. I could only think of religious images of Jesus and saints walking effortlessly on the clouds on the way to Heaven.

Before I knew it, the flight attendant placed a tray in front of each of us. I saw a small white cup. I lifted it to my mouth, taking a cautious sip. The taste was completely unfamiliar, and I almost vomited, not knowing what that strange liquid was. I immediately spat the contents of my mouth back into the cup. I noticed that Costy was watching me, and I told him I had never tasted anything like that in my life, so he did not even deign to lift his cup to his mouth. Only later would I learn that this was cold milk, something I cannot drink to this day unless it is drowning in chocolate. I cannot remember any other conversations with my brother. Did we sleep during the flight? I cannot say for sure, but I suspect we must have dozed on and off.

Much to our surprise, the plane stopped in Rotterdam, and we were taken in hand by the airline staff as soon as we reached the gate. Our papers were checked, and somehow, it seemed, we had missed some vaccination or other before leaving Lebanon. So we were duly escorted to a nurse's station and given shots. Costy and I were both ill at ease, and we exchanged few words, but I always held onto his hand, never letting him out of my sight, lest someone kidnap us to fill our bellies with drugs.

It seemed like we sat alone in a tiny room forever before a flight attendant arrived and escorted us onto another plane, this one headed to New York. We were once again seated in the back, well within the watchful eyes of the KLM crew. When the next meal was served, both my brother and I were cautious about dipping our utensils into the food. Fortunately, there was bread, and we both ate that.

Costy and I exchanged few words. I suspect we were both in some altered state. Soon enough, the captain announced that we would be landing in Idlewild Airport in New York. The flight attendant made sure our seat belts were buckled, and Costy and I looked at each other as the plane pressure changed. I noticed that his hands were grabbing his seat as mine were clutching my own seat.

***

The plane stopped in the middle of a large, empty cement area. The attendant told me in French that we should sit until the other passengers had deplaned. I told Costy in Arabic, and we had nothing to do but stare at the people walking from the bottom of the stairs to the terminal on our left. Our turn to deplane came faster than we expected. The flight attendant took each of us by the hand. She spoke to us in French, but I found myself too curious to pay attention, instead directing my eyes at the other passengers walking in front of us, as though we were all in some strange parade with two children bringing up the rear.

Soon enough, we were inside the terminal, with the flight attendant giving us an enormous smile. "*Nous voilà,*" (here we are) she said, gazing at a group of people standing with enormous cards bearing our names. The attendant exchanged words with my uncle, whom I remembered from Lebanon, and handed us over to him and his family.

My uncle—tall, balding, and more athletic than my father—took our hands and proceeded to walk away from the attendant. Examining our tickets, he spotted the luggage tags. He called out to the attendant, who graciously approached him. He asked her with an aggressive voice what those things were. I could not understand the words, but the hand gestures told me all I needed to know.

My uncle went into a state of fury, screaming at me and Costy. Neither of us understood a word of the sentences flying out of his mouth, nor could we understand what the flight attendant was answering in English. Only later would I learn that he had given strict orders to Mama Hana to send the children alone and without any luggage, orders she and Aunt Najla had obviously ignored.

Years later, I can see the almost comical absurdity of my uncle's yelling at us in a language we did not understand (a fact of which he was well aware). The decision not to use his and our native tongue, the Lebanese dialect of Arabic, may have partly resulted from the irrationality of his fury. But I think, more fundamentally, it was part of my uncle's project to scrub the smell of the old country out of us as quickly as possible.

Before I knew it, he had grabbed our hands again and started walking in enormous steps toward the luggage area, words spewing out of his mouth all the while. Neither his wife Olga nor his other children let out a peep. Their wordless passivity made me think of sheep in the village being led to slaughter. The other passengers had long since disappeared with their luggage, leaving only one suitcase, one of ours. My uncle looked at the tags again and suddenly realized that the other suitcase had not arrived. The flight attendant had meanwhile disappeared, and the luggage staff had made themselves scarce. My uncle pulled Costy and me into the KLM office and proceeded to yell at the staff. I dared not look at Costy, but I suspect he was as frightened as I was. I wanted to disappear but could not. I prayed that an angel would take me and Costy by the hand and fly us away. But that was not to be. The staff did manage to stop my uncle from screaming. As to their conversation, I could not understand a word.

The next thing I knew, Costy and I were being dragged by my uncle's long strides toward a parking lot, followed by the rest of the family and the lone suitcase. We were placed in the back seat of a blue car, squeezed between cousins. My aunt took the front seat, with another cousin sitting between her and Michel, whose hands firmly gripped the wheel.

Our journey to the promised land had begun. My uncle started driving away, with the enormous solitary suitcase in the trunk. Did he stop screaming? I do not remember. I do remember feeling isolated, lonely, and lost. I forced myself to think about Lebanon. I could hear a conversation in the car but had no idea what was being said. Things became slightly clearer when my uncle pulled into the parking lot of a diner and everyone exited the car. We were escorted inside and seated between family members. I looked at my brother, and he seemed as clueless as I was.

The noise in the crowded diner reminded me of a shop in a Beirut *souk*. At last, a woman arrived at the table wearing an apron and, pad in hand, began writing I know not what. Before long, plates buried under food began arriving at the table. A large dish was placed in front of me. It was brimming with what looked like spaghetti, except the strands were thicker than the ones I was accustomed to in Lebanon. The long, thick, white threads of pasta were drowning in a bright red sauce topped with little balls bathed in the same thick red liquid. The waitress also placed baskets of what must have been bread. It did not look at all like the bread we were used to.

I watched as family members around the long table began grabbing pieces of bread and spreading some yellowish paste on it. None of it looked familiar. Neither my brother nor I made a move toward the food. Suddenly, my uncle, who was facing me across the table, began screaming. I could not understand a word he said, but he was clearly furious. He made motions with his hands, indicating that Costy and I should eat. To me, the food was both alien and unappetizing, and the massive size of the American portion made it even more threatening. I immediately began to cry. Constantine expressed his defiance by pushing the plate away. In a flash, my uncle, seated next to my brother, delivered a resounding blow to the back of his head. I have no memory of the rest of the meal, except that both my brother and I were in tears. I believe I ate some of the spaghetti and meatballs; whether Costy ate anything at all, I have no idea.

***

Eventually, we arrived in Ithaca, New York and at my uncle's house: 418 Mitchell Street, an address I will never forget. Costy and I were taken inside, while my uncle emptied the trunk of the car with the help of his son, George—a tall, fit young man with dark hair who emerged from the house. My uncle began shouting again, but I could not cover my ears, so I started humming French and Arabic tunes in my head.

I had already noticed that "The House of Horror," as I would later dub it, was nowhere near the size of our house in Deir el-Amar. It stood silently on a street, surrounded by what were clearly its cousins: houses of the same shape and size but painted different dull colors: beige, light brown, yellow, and white.

Soon, everyone sat down in the living room while my aunt Olga, a mature, slightly overweight woman with thin, dusty reddish-blonde hair, went to the kitchen. She returned with a large tray, holding empty glasses and a pitcher of water. She walked around the living room, offering each of us a glass of water.

I took one and drank slowly. I looked at Costy, who did the same. Meanwhile the large suitcase and our two KLM bags had been placed in an adjoining small rectangular room next to the stairs leading to the upper floors.

It was already fairly late, and my brother and I were obviously exhausted. The decision about where the two of us would sleep had already been made. This was far from *The Sound of Music*, and my brother and I did not perform for the family before being whisked off to bed. Costy shared the bed in George's room, and I would sleep in the bed with Connie, Michel's youngest (and most beautiful) daughter, whose room was adjacent to that of her brother. We were given pajamas, and our travel clothing was whisked away. I know that I fell asleep from exhaustion as soon as my head hit the pillow, with Connie by my side. I suspect Costy did the same, but with George at his side.

The next day began inauspiciously. Olga had gone up to the attic and brought down used clothing for me and Costy to wear. I was put in a short-sleeved faded navy-blue dress that I can still see vividly in front of me. I do not remember what Costy wore, but it was most likely a used pair of pants and a shirt. Gone were the brand-new European-style clothes from Beirut (along with the beautiful blue suitcases angrily discarded by my uncle), replaced by American hand-me-downs.

CHAPTER 15

Family Rituals

I remember little about daily events from that time. Only a few significant memories still occupy my brain. One morning, Olga's brother, Uncle Herb, and his wife, Aunt Helen, had arrived at the house and were awaiting us. It must have been Sunday, because we were going to church. Absent from the outing was Michel, who, I later learned, boycotted church on principle, as well as George and Connie, Michel and Olga's two youngest. Both studying at Cornell at the time, George and Connie still lived in the family house. The other children, now adults, had moved on.

I remember Aunt Helen at the bottom of the stairs, watching me come down and taking me aside. She scrutinized me from head to toe. She rubbed her hands on my legs and somehow made it clear to me that I had hair on them and that this was unacceptable. The name of Connie came up, and I deduced from that that Connie would be in charge of teaching me how to groom myself appropriately. If I say that I have never had much hair on my legs, I run the risk of sounding defensive, but it happens to be the truth. Aunt Helen also pointed, with appropriate facial gestures, to the sweat stains on the armpits of my short-sleeved dress (we did not use deodorant in Lebanon). The message stuck: everything about me was wrong. I did not look right. I smelled bad. To this day, I go to elaborate lengths to cover my body with expensive perfumes and scented lotions.

The details escape me now, but the larger image is still there. We were all heading to church. When we arrived, Olga duly introduced us to the smiling minister who was greeting worshippers at the door. When I set eyes on the church, I was shocked. When I first learned we were going to church, I was delighted. For me, a church was a beautiful building with graceful arches and glorious masonry, stained glass windows, colorful Stations of the Cross, paintings of the Virgin Mary, a large cross on the altar to which the body of Christ was nailed, and perhaps, here and there, a statue of a saint. I had grown accustomed to hearing church bells ring to welcome worshippers and to being immersed in clouds of incense. I found myself in, however, what I can only describe as a sterile space. Sure, there were benches for worshippers to slide into, which is precisely what we did. The service began, and I understood not a word. I was actually grateful when it was over and we went back to Mitchell Street.

Costy and I were put in charge of cleaning the house, washing the dishes, and doing chores—something that made me realize I had grown up in a privileged environment in Lebanon, where Umm Zahiyya took care of such tasks. Connie and George, though living with us, had no household duties I was aware of. Had they helped out when they were younger? I have no way of knowing.

My uncle always sat on the couch in the living room watching television while we were cleaning. I can still hear Lawrence Welk's "a one, and a two, and a three" before he would engage his orchestra. I do not believe that my uncle ever missed an episode of that show. I was not bothered by having to vacuum the house or get down on my knees to wipe the kitchen and bathroom floors. Sometimes, I would find coins on the floor or in the upholstery that I would slip into my pockets. Neither Costy nor I received an allowance. Nor did we expect one, for that was not a Lebanese custom.

My brother and I were also in charge of cleaning up after meals: clearing the table as well as washing the dirty dishes, pots, and pans. I would dip my bare hands in the hot sink water and scrub the dirt and then rinse the utensils. Costy stood by my side with a towel in his hands, ready to dry the clean dinnerware and cookware.

During these tasks, we would stand next to each other in front of the sink, with the kitchen and dining room behind us. We would speak furtively to each other in Arabic because we had no other language in which to express ourselves. Olga came by once and heard us speaking to one another and, of course, could not understand what we were saying. I had not been vigilant and did not realize she was standing behind us.

Suddenly, I heard my aunt speaking to us. She was furious, and she began explaining in English very slowly to make sure we understood that if she ever caught us speaking Arabic or French, she would tell our dad, who would then beat us, for we were forbidden to speak anything other than English under pain of physical punishment.

Decades later, I was speaking to a psychiatrist about my childhood, and she explained to me that if someone like my uncle Michel beat me and my brother, he would not have begun such behavior late in life. Rather, he must have beaten others before we set foot on the stage, and that his victims likely included his wife

Olga. So what my aunt was doing that day in the kitchen, besides being complicit and an enabler of my uncle's cruelty, was protecting herself. If Michel took out his sadism on me and my brother, he need not take it out on my aunt Olga.

We were told to call my uncle Michel "Dad," and his wife Olga "Mother." The word *Dad* was totally alien to both of us, but we just went along.

***

There are scenes that play and replay in my mind and that I am incapable of exorcising. One day, not long after our arrival, Connie expressed her admiration for three thin gold bangles I wore on my right arm: one was a gift from Aunt Najla, and the other two came from Mama Hana's arm, part of a set Papa had offered her on the occasion of their marriage.

I had grown up in a culture that dictated that when someone offered a compliment on something you were wearing or carrying, you would thank them and then offer the object. Middle Eastern politeness then dictated that the other person would decline the offer and repeat the compliment.

So when Connie complimented me on my gold bangles, I began performing the appropriate ritual, offering her the bracelets. Much to my consternation, she slipped the bangles off my right arm and placed them on hers. Then she began re-admiring the gold jewelry, but this time on her own arm while she twirled it around and moved the bangles up and down. I did not know what to say or how to respond to what to me was not merely a clear act of impoliteness, but an appropriation of what had become part of my body. I felt violated. I headed to the bathroom just across from Connie's room and began to cry. Gone were the gifts from Aunt Najla and Mama Hana. My arm felt naked, and I felt as if I had lost a part of myself.

Connie wore the bangles happily, making sure to show them to every member of the family who complimented her, adding how beautiful she looked with the gold shining on her arm. Fortunately, a few years later, Connie, whose bed I still shared, became bored with the gold bracelets and returned them to me. I merely thanked her without further ado.

Did I share this experience with my brother Costy? I do not remember. I suspect I was much too upset. Instead of bringing us together, the forbidding climate of my uncle's house gradually distanced us from each other.

***

The episode with the gold bangles cannot even come close to the scene that plays and replays in my mind like an endless horror movie. This film comprises the beatings to which Costy was subjected. My uncle would place my brother face down on the living room coffee table. Then he would go outside and pull a knotted branch off one of the trees in the back yard. When he returned, branch in his right hand, he would pull my brother's pants and underwear down to his knees and start hitting him over and over on his behind with the knotted branch. I stood looking in horror through the kitchen door as fresh red blood oozed out of my brother's buttocks. My uncle would begin yelling and screaming, calling Costy "*Manhous*," as he lifted the tree branch in his strong right arm and brought it down on my brother's pink behind.

Now that I relive these beating episodes in my mind, I can see my uncle's face as he screamed "*Manhous*" over and over again, while his arm rose and then landed on my brother's bleeding flesh. I realize in retrospect that he was, during these beatings, like a man possessed, pulse racing, heart beating wildly.

"*Manhous*," in Arabic, means he who is unlucky or brings bad luck to people. There is a proverb that says "*al-manhous bi-yehuttu ala ra'su fanous*," which means that people put a lamp (*fanous*) on the *manhous*'s head so they can see him coming and avoid him. *Manhous* became Costy's name for the entire time I lived in my uncle's house.

During these beatings, somehow my aunt Olga, aka Mother, would disappear into the air like a genie from the *Arabian Nights*. I would then run down to the basement, walk silently past a brick wall on my left, and stop for a few moments. My young imagination would begin madly racing as I found myself in the Poe short story, "The Cask of Amontillado." Hammer in hand, in my fantasy, I would smash the wall, throw my uncle behind it, and let him scream while I sealed the wall behind me.

In the real-life horror story, however, I continued through the basement to the opposite side, where there were enormous barrels filled with apples. I would grab an apple, stuff it into my mouth, core and all (to leave no telltale remnants), barely chewing it, then grab another apple, once again stuffing it into my mouth, then another and another and another. I never took too many apples from the same barrel, lest my aunt Olga discover that one barrel was missing apples when she came down to collect the fruit for an apple pie. But I could not block my brother's loud screams, and I imagined the blood flowing from his body while I swallowed one apple after another.

A cold floor my couch,
    I stare at the wall.
    Edgar Allen Poe
    Serenading me.
He already knows
My favorite tale
As his southern voice
Takes me to oblivion.

Eventually, the screams would die down, and I always assumed this was a signal that the beating had stopped. I would quietly climb the stairs that led to the kitchen door and sneak back into the kitchen. I always attempted a peek into the living room before going any further. I could see my uncle sitting, spent and slightly dazed, on the couch. In front of him, the coffee table on which he was wont to stretch his legs was now marred by my brother's blood. Constantine was nowhere to be seen. I assumed that he went to the room he shared with George and covered himself up. I dashed upstairs myself, as Michel called his wife to clean the table. My mind still echoed (as it does even today) with Aunt Najla's admonition that I must protect my younger brother, but I could do nothing. I was helpless with rage, humiliation, and guilt.

At that time, Costy loved the color green. With the coins I had collected while cleaning the floors, I would run out of the house and walk to downtown Ithaca, which was not very far. I would purchase lime lifesavers, wrapped in green, and quickly return to the house. When I had a quiet moment, I would slip the lifesavers to my brother as a gift. We never discussed the beatings.

My uncle's hands did not spare me. But as an Arab male, he could not do to me what he did to Costy—that is, take down my underwear and strike my naked body. Instead, his strong arm always landed on my neck, shoulders, and back. I felt great pain and also cried and screamed, but I would never dream of comparing my beatings to what Costy underwent on a regular basis. These beatings were never discussed in the Malti family. They were simply a part of daily existence. I do remember that one day George, who was living in the house while attending Cornell Law School, came down to complain that the noise was distracting him from his studying. How did Michel react? I have no memory, but I do know that the beatings continued.

Sometimes, when I describe Constantine's ordeal, listeners ask, "But what had Constantine done to provoke such punishment?" I have trouble bringing myself to answer because, to me, no transgression could justify such brutality. But the answer, incredible as it may seem to some who have lived sheltered lives, is that Constantine did not do anything. Neither Costy nor I were overtly rebellious (we were much too scared). My brother did not steal. He did not curse. He did not break things. He never hit anyone. He did not run away. To this day I am amazed that Constantine, despite all he has gone through, has become such a gentle and compassionate man. If Constantine had a fault—if this is a fault—it was that he did not do well in school. But I was beaten, too, though not as severely, and I was always a model student.

***

Costy and I had arrived in America in August, and the school year was to begin soon. To determine the grade in which we should be placed, we took written exams. We both could barely navigate the everyday English to which we were exposed. When I was asked a question, I would simply answer "Yes" or "No" depending, literally, on my mood. Having arrived in America with nary a word of English, it was no surprise that we both flunked the exams miserably. It did not matter. We were both assigned to grades with students below our respective ages. I felt humiliated because I had always been a star pupil in Lebanon, but that was of no use here. In any case, we had no choice. We were bit players in a drama whose language we barely understood.

I remember very little of my education in Ithaca. Only a few events stick out from what was to me an alien environment. We were asked to write a two-page short story for an English class, and the best one would be read aloud. I worked very hard with my limited English to write a story about a prisoner in a small triangular room with cement walls, enormously tall but of different heights. The room had a tiny, barred window on the highest part of the pitched ceiling. The prisoner had to bend his neck to see any light from that small window. He was to be executed the next day, and he spent the night staring at whatever little bit of sky he could see. The story ended as dawn was rising and guards were knocking on the cell door to take the prisoner to be hanged.

I confess that I was very proud of my story as I handed it in to the teacher. Much to my shock, the teacher chose another student to present her story to the class. I sat and listened to the student read what to me was a ridiculous tale about a boy who liked a girl in his school, so he decided to pick some flowers and place them in a bouquet. Then he worked up the courage to walk to her house, climb the front steps, and ring the doorbell. The girl opened the door, and he offered her the bouquet as she blushed.

This was the winning story: a budding romance, appropriate for our stage of life and ending on a sweet note. I remember this event as though it were yesterday. I got my story back with no comments from the teacher; there may have been signs of a missing comma here or there, but I cannot remember. Much later in life, I shared this event with Allen, and he was not surprised the other story was chosen. My story was too dark for someone my age, it seems.

What I long forgot about were the cheap tabloids that my uncle would buy on weekends. They were sold, folded in three, presumably to hide the garish black-and-white photographs from newsstand gawkers or vulnerable children. He would read them and throw them out. I would then retrieve them and attempt to read them. They contained illustrated true-crime stories about murders, break-ins, rapes, and the like. At the time, I could barely understand them.

Junior high school meant taking the school bus daily. Most of the time, I sat alone near a window. But then, one day, toward the end of the school year, I was surprised to see a male African American student sit next to me. My English was still weak, and I do not believe he and I exchanged a single word. After sitting next to me a few times, he got his courage up and took one of my hands in his. I did not move to stop him. Instead I found myself mesmerized by his hand. It fascinated me because unlike my own hand, it seemed to have more than one color. The top of the hand was brown, the color of his face. But when he turned his hand to grab mine, the palm of his hand was pink. I would stare and stare at this wondrous color combination. I believe that he got off the bus before I did, but I cannot be sure. What I was certain about was that if my Uncle Michel had an inkling of this, I would have been beaten mercilessly. I never mentioned this seating arrangement to anyone, though other students must have noticed it.

***

I mumbled and stumbled through junior high school. In my first year in the school, I got my first phone call. The phone was in a little room on the first floor next to the stairs. When it rang, my aunt picked it up and then called me. The voice on the phone had asked for me by name. Both Connie and George had appeared in the little room, hoping the call was for them.

When my aunt handed me the phone, everyone stood still. I said "Hello," and the male voice on the other end of the line said something and hung up. I stood there as everyone was questioning me. What did the person say to Fedwa? I repeated the words I had heard: "Fuck you." Everyone stared at me in horror. I almost felt like I was being suspected of witchcraft.

I was bombarded with questions. Who was the caller? Did I recognize the voice? Why would this individual call me and say such a thing? My uncle heard the ruckus and joined the party. He screamed at me:

"What did you do, you stupid girl?"

"Nothing," I answered.

Raising his right arm, he began beating me on the neck, the shoulders, and the back, insisting with each blow that no one gets calls like that without a reason. As his beatings continued, I began to cry. My aunt tried to calm him down, but he quickly shut her up.

"You are nothing but a *sharmouta*, just like your mother," he was now screaming at me as his arm landed again and again on my neck and shoulders. I stood still as a statue as his words assaulted my ears. I had graduated from being a "stupid girl" to a "*sharmouta*." My new title would follow me throughout my life as long as my uncle was alive.

"*Sharmouta*." I knew growing up in Lebanon that this was a very bad word that one should never use. It means a whore, a prostitute, a loose woman, and a host of other disgusting connotations that have to do with street women who sell their bodies. I should not have been shocked hearing this word exit my uncle's mouth. After all, had not Costy become "*Manhous?*" That I should become "*Sharmouta*" was a natural linguistic parallel, except for its sexual connotations. My American family did not know what these two words meant nor would they have dared to ask my uncle. Besides, these were the only two Arabic words I ever heard him utter.

CHAPTER 16

The Attic

School was a welcome change from the atmosphere at home, even though for the first few years I did not understand all that was taught. Much of the learning simply flew by me, like a lost bird looking for its nest. Our instruction in junior high school included French. The class was on an elementary level, but I was still not accustomed to speaking in class.

One day, the teacher called on me, and I responded in perfect French. She held me up as an example to the other students that it was possible to mimic her, as I had done so perfectly. After weeks of French classes in which I always seemed to have the correct answer when called upon, she took me aside after class and began questioning me. Why was it that my French was so good, she wanted to know?

At the time, I always tried to make myself invisible. My clothing all came from the attic in the house. By the time I wore that clothing, it had seen several generations of cousins, since my uncle had five daughters and only one son. It goes without saying that there were no uniforms in American public schools at the time, as opposed to what I had grown up with in Catholic boarding schools.

When the French teacher's questioning began, I was frightened. The last thing I wanted was to be subjected to more beatings because of something inappropriate I might have done, such as answering questions in perfect French. I attempted to evade the questions, which was not too difficult since the teacher was speaking to me in English, and I was never completely sure of understanding her. She finally decided to question me in French, and I shuddered. I could no longer play the game my way. I had to answer in French. The teacher started probing slowly and then more deeply as she began to realize that I was fluent in French.

I expected anger on her part, something to which I had become accustomed in the home environment. Instead, she smiled at me and began a long conversation in French. She asked me about the nuns in Lebanon, about my experience as a boarder, and about what I had been taught. I was embarrassed. Since our arrival in America, no one had ever taken such an interest, either in me or in my former education.

She insisted on accompanying me to my uncle's house, since the school buses had long gone. I sat in her car, overwhelmed by fear. What would my uncle say? I was late and had missed the school bus. I was sure to get a beating. Soon we were in front of my uncle's house. My teacher insisted on accompanying me inside.

I was shaking as she rang the doorbell, and my uncle opened the door. He was shocked to see the young woman standing next to me. The teacher introduced herself and began to explain the reasons for my delay, so he finally invited her into the house. Olga, realizing there was a guest, rushed out of the kitchen, introduced herself, and offered a cold drink. At this point, I was completely lost. I expected my uncle to scream, but he was on his best behavior. The teacher accepted the drink gracefully and sat on the couch with my uncle. Before I knew it, my cousin George had appeared and introduced himself to her.

I had retreated to a corner between the living room and dining room where no one would pay attention to me. George, on the other hand, began a long conversation with my French teacher, and the two seemed quite comfortable with one another. I continued to retreat, first to the dining room and then to the kitchen, where I sat in the empty breakfast nook. My aunt Olga had not reappeared, so I assumed that she was with the others in the living room.

Some time passed, and then I heard my uncle's voice calling me in an unfamiliar tone: soft, lacking anger. I made my way to the living room, where everyone seemed at ease. My French teacher was getting ready to leave, and I could sense that she and George would see one another again. Even my uncle looked pleased. My teacher said her goodbyes and left. I stood there, feeling like an extra in a drama that had played itself out without me. My uncle told me to go to my room now, something I was only too happy to do. Nothing was said about my performance in school or my language skills. The beating I expected never materialized.

Only now, writing these pages, do I understand that my uncle knew how to mask his temper when dealing with people outside the family. One does not become a professor in an Ivy League university without some skill in hiding one's demons. The happy result of this incident was that I was now permitted to spend French classes in the back of the room, devouring French literature. French was my companion again and has remained my close friend to this day. Arabic would take much longer to reconquer.

***

One night, Connie arrived home very late, long after I had fallen asleep. She woke me and started speaking very fast. She smelled of alcohol, and I was not sure what she was saying. She decided we should go down to the kitchen. I was a bit surprised, but I followed her and watched as she took a box of chocolate cake mix and started preparing the mixture. We then had a bowl of chocolate cake mix. I thought she was going to put it in the oven, but instead, she opened the silverware drawer, grabbed two spoons, and handed me one. I stared as she dipped the spoon into the mixture and began eating it raw. She urged me to do the same. I found it delicious.

Giggling, Connie started up the stairs, beckoning me to follow her, and we headed for her bedroom at the end of the hall and crawled into bed with the bowl of doughy chocolate mix between us. Then she started talking to me about the fraternity party she had just attended at Cornell and said that she had been raped. I was not sure what all this meant, and my confused face must have given me away. She explained everything at least twice more until I believe I understood. She talked most of the night, and at last, we fell asleep, bellies full of chocolate cake mix.

The next day led to a new exile. Olga and Michel had discovered our nightly adventure, and there was hell to pay. Connie was chastised lightly—I never saw my uncle hit any of his own children, though he may have when they were younger. My aunt and uncle decided that Constantine and I should be moved to the attic and no longer share beds with Connie and George.

The attic had been used as storage space, but by moving boxes around, my aunt and uncle managed to find two small areas where Costy and I could sleep on mattresses on the floor. To access the stairs leading to the attic, my brother and I had to go through Michel and Olga's bedroom. There was also no bathroom, so we had to go down the stairs to the second floor to use the toilet or wash ourselves, each time crossing my aunt and uncle's bedroom, where they slept in separate beds.

***

One morning, I awoke in the attic with a wet, sticky feeling in my underwear. I dared not say a word to my brother, so I snuck out of the room, headed for a dark corner in the hallway, and pulled my underpants down. Bright red blood covered my underwear and blood that was still flowing out of my body. I was horrified and certain I was going to die.

I returned to the room, where Costy was still asleep, and crawled back under my covers. I closed my eyes to make it look like I was still asleep, but an earthquake was shaking my head so hard I was sure it would break into pieces. Why me? I prayed like a mad woman, but I could still feel that yucky blood. Constantine, meanwhile, had awakened and gotten dressed. I was still feigning sleep as he headed downstairs, most likely to use the bathroom.

I felt like my entire world had fallen on top of me. The only person with whom I felt I could share this strange secret was Connie, but to reach her, I had to go through my uncle and aunt's bedroom. I looked at the clock and prayed that they would be downstairs having their breakfast. I moved quietly down the stairs, through their bedroom, and quickly entered Connie's room.

She was awake but still in bed. She looked at me strangely and could probably tell I was upset. She invited me to sit on her bed, which I did. Then she asked me what was wrong. I felt myself struggling to get out the words, and much to my shock, Connie began to smile. I wanted to scream, but nothing came out of my throat. She explained to me that I was experiencing my first period, that I should expect this event once a month and that this was perfectly normal. Much to my surprise, Connie then gave me a hug and accompanied me to the bathroom.

I cleaned myself while she opened the large bathroom closet that held towels and handed me what I later learned was a Kotex. She showed me how to use it and then advised me to go back upstairs, change my underwear, rinse the old pair, take a new pair, and do what she had shown me to do with the Kotex. Once that new one became full of blood, I was to simply roll it tight, wrap it in toilet paper, and throw it in the garbage. Then she laughed and said that as far as she knew, there had always been Kotex in that closet. After all, had she not grown up in a house with four sisters? The secret we had shared would remain between us, she added, as she hugged me. I was overwhelmed with relief.

***

Our first summer in Ithaca, Costy and I were sent to a summer camp while my uncle and his wife took a vacation. The camp was on a lake, and Olga had packed me some clothing, including an old swimsuit from the attic. I shared a cabin with other girls; whether it was two or three, I cannot remember. I found the entire experience rather strange. Perhaps Costy and I should have been grateful for this camp experience, which at least gave us a respite from my uncle's heavy hand.

We learned only later that my uncle regretted spending the money on the camp, and the subsequent summers while we lived in Ithaca, we were sent to live with Michel's married daughters.

We spent one summer in Massachusetts (if my memory is correct) with the oldest daughter, Helen, and her husband Lee, a Methodist preacher. What I am certain of is that the couple was overjoyed to have us, turning us into indentured servants. I do not believe this is an exaggeration. They had an enormous amount of land with a lawn and a flower garden. Costy and I were forced to spend our days in the hot sun on our knees, pulling weeds.

It was not simply the sun beating down on our heads that made the task unpleasant. It was also the threats. Helen's husband, Lee, gave each of us a metal pot to collect the weeds. Lee would come around regularly and glance at the pots (emptying them as necessary) to monitor our progress. We were told that if we did not pick enough weeds, we would be deprived of food that day. I do not remember speaking to Costy much on these occasions. What I do remember was being afraid and trying not to cry. Maybe this was good character training, but it did not feel that way to me.

At odd times, that summer, I know for certain that while pulling weeds, my thoughts would wander to Lebanon and to the farm our family owned. How free I remembered feeling, as Costy and I would walk through the grass, each of us holding one of Papa's hands with one of ours. Here we were, this time, backs bent, pulling weeds to earn our supper.

***

We returned to Ithaca in time for school. The routine of Constantine's beatings continued along with my escape to the basement. My brother and I never spoke of these events. Were we too frightened, or just numb?

Aunt Najla sent Costy and me letters in her broken English telling us to obey our uncle. After all, she would repeat over and over, what a generous act it was on his part to adopt the two of us and take on the burden of raising two children after his were already grown. At times, she would add bits of news about people in the village. I read her missives carefully, but gradually I began to feel as if she were writing about another planet. I do not remember responding to any of her letters. What would I write? That my brother and I had somehow landed in Hell while still alive? That we had been exiled to the attic? All that would mean nothing to her.

***

I was now in my last year of Junior High. I could feel the excitement among the students but did not understand its cause. As the school year progressed, I learned that we would all be moving on to High School. And to celebrate this transition, there would be a prom at the end of the year. Conversations revolved around this important event. Would a girl be invited? Who would invite her? I am not sure how much book learning went on that year.

I was invited to the prom. Who invited me? The son of the director of the leading funeral home in Ithaca. My first reaction was astonishment. The coincidence of the son of a funeral home director asking me to the prom weighed heavily on my mind. Why a funeral director's son? I was overwhelmed with morbidity, something I had lived with from the moment my father died.

The family was excited. Fedwa's date was considered hot property, since his father was such a successful businessman. What I would wear was the big question. Everyone became involved as dresses, already worn by different cousins, were dragged out of the attic and brought to Michel and Olga's bedroom, where there was a mirror. I would try on a dress, and my audience would vote yes or no. Every dress seemed to have a problem. One might be torn, another would be too small, yet another would be too large. I played along with this charade because it was clear that my uncle was not about to purchase a new prom dress for the *sharmouta*.

I remember feeling depressed by the process of putting on a dress and taking it off, then putting on another dress and taking it off, then putting on a third and fourth and fifth dress. There was obviously something wrong with my body. My modeling continued as more and more dresses appeared only to disappear after I tried them on: too long, too short, too tight, too large.

Finally, my female audience settled on a dress. It had short sleeves, a zipper in the back, and fit me reasonably well. The only problem was that its age was showing, and no one could remember to which Malti girl it had belonged. It had clearly never been worn by Connie, but that left Alice, Emily, Ruth, and Helen, Helen being the oldest of the children.

This to-be prom dress was made of taffeta. Its original pink had faded to an orange hue, but this color was not consistent throughout the dress. Parts of it were more pink than others, and I recognized the odor of old clothing from my younger days in Lebanon when Aunt Najla would rummage around the piles of clothing hidden behind the large curtain in her room. No matter. The problem of

Fedwa's dress was solved. I was not asked if I was happy with the dress. All anyone cared about was that I would blissfully cost nothing for this school ritual.

One problem remained, however: shoes. High heels were a must at a prom. The dresses not chosen returned to their home in the attic. Instead, their companions, high-heeled shoes, made their descent to the second floor. There I was, once again, but this time seated. I found myself slipping my feet into shoes that had lived for years alongside those dresses in the attic. Slipping high-heeled shoes on and off was painful on my feet, especially if the shoes were too tight, which most of them were. If not too tight, they would be too large. None of the high-heeled shoes fit my feet. Olga and Connie, my two helpers, gave my uncle the bad news.

As usual, he began screaming at me. Not only was I a *sharmouta*, but I was going to cost him money because I needed high-heeled shoes for the prom. Up to that time, Costy and I had been able to find clothing and shoes from the attic, but heels were another matter. Connie, her parents' darling, took up my cause and managed to calm her father. She would take me shopping for the cheapest high heels we could find, she reassured Michel.

Sure enough, Connie took me shopping. And, miraculously, she found an inexpensive pair of pink high heels that fit my feet. I realized in the store that the pink shoes did not match the faded color of the dress. I said nothing to Connie about it. Perhaps she had not noticed. But I did not feel comfortable discussing my problem with her. I knew she would laugh it off. I resigned myself to looking mismatched. The irony of my teen-aged desolation is that today, I would be delighted—stunned, even—to be able to wear high heels at all.

The day of the prom, I realized that I really did not want to go. I felt ill at ease the whole day, knowing that I had no choice. When the doorbell rang that evening, I was filled with a sense of doom. My date was at the door and was greeted by the entire family. He stepped into the house and pinned a corsage on my dress. My fate was sealed; I had to go to the prom. The young man's father was awaiting us in a dark sedan. I slipped into the back seat, and my date sat next to me. The inside of the car was black, just like the outside. I was ashamed of the new shoes that did not match the old dress and silently cursed my fate.

I felt, rightly or wrongly, that I was haunted by death. As the car started moving, I caught myself doing what we girls used to do in boarding school in Lebanon, trying to recreate the smell of death. I was certain that the odor of death pervaded the car. Papa's demise was foremost in my mind as we arrived at the prom. I remember nothing else about this event, which to me became intertwined with dying. I must not have been a very cheerful date.

CHAPTER 17

Florida

The prom ended my days in Ithaca. Before I knew it, my aunt and uncle were talking about packing up and driving to Miami, Florida. Florida? This came as a complete surprise. Had I been living in a cocoon, oblivious to everything going on around me? Apparently, while I was buried in my own world, my uncle had reached retirement age at Cornell and had been offered a position at the University of Miami in Coral Gables. The family would be moving to Miami. Not only that, but my uncle had even purchased a house with a canal behind it in a nice area of Miami.

Connie, meanwhile, had become pregnant after her date rape, and it was decided that she would stay with Alice and her husband on their farm in Munnsville, New York. Costy and I had spent part of a summer there, and it was much more restful than the summer with Helen and her husband. I remember Costy was quite excited when he had a chance to ride a tractor. I spent the time helping Alice around the house and reading. I will never forget that summer because that was when I read *Lady Chatterly's Lover*.

All I knew about Florida was that Connie had spent a spring break there. A photographer spotted her in her bathing suit and took a photograph of her leaning against a palm tree, if I remember correctly. The photo, featured in a newspaper, was cut out and pasted on the refrigerator door in the Malti kitchen in Ithaca. Connie was quite beautiful, and no one seemed surprised to see her posed in a swimsuit on the refrigerator.

***

In preparation for the car trip to Florida, I helped in the kitchen while my aunt Olga baked an endless collection of cookies and brownies (with and without nuts), made a basketful of sandwiches, and loaded the car with fruit. Costy and I each packed a small suitcase placed alongside other small suitcases for my aunt and uncle in the trunk of the car.

My uncle decided that he would drive from Ithaca to Miami. He had mapped out everything in advance. As a more experienced traveler, I now recognize that, back in 1962, the journey could easily have required between twenty-four and thirty hours on the road, making only minimum stops for gas or traffic. Did my uncle plan this for one long push? I do not remember stopping for the night. My brother, however, says we spent one night in a motel.

Despite being in his late sixties, my uncle was confident he could accomplish this drive easily. He had had the car checked out and filled it with gas, and the morning of departure came faster than any of us anticipated. I was personally excited about a change, and the picture of Connie on the refrigerator told me that the scenery would at least be different from that of upstate New York.

The day of departure came. My brother and I sat next to one another in the back seat of the car alongside the food. We were in charge of passing whatever package Olga requested to her in the front seat. There was also bottled water, in case anyone became thirsty.

We set out at dawn and, hours later, were on an unlit two-lane highway at night. Suddenly, the car headed off the highway to the right and literally flew in the air before landing in the midst of trees. I remember thinking we were about to die and silently reciting to myself all the prayers I had learned in boarding school. No one said a word. This was before the day of cell phones, so my uncle could not call for help. I have forgotten completely how we managed to get out of that spot.

My mind goes blank on the rest of the trip until we arrived in the state of Florida with its "Welcome to Florida" signs, replete with pictures of oranges. I seem to recall my uncle parking the car and ordering us all to get out and follow him to one of the buildings. We went inside the enormous room filled with travel pamphlets. Stands offered free orange juice, and each of us received a glass. The people were friendly and smiling, as they welcomed us to Florida.

I still remember the taste of that juice: delicately sweet and incredibly refreshing. I sipped it as slowly as I could, savoring every drop that graced my tongue. How different it tasted from the frozen orange juice that my aunt Olga served at breakfast in Ithaca. Had we somehow landed in Paradise? I could not help but think of Lebanon and the delicious tangerines. I had to hold back the tears from my eyes, knowing only too well that were my uncle to spot my emotional state, I would be in for a beating. Soon, my reverie was broken by his voice. "Come on, come on, come on," he bellowed. Whatever fantasy world I was in came to an end as we all piled back into the car.

My uncle had apparently purchased a house in Miami. When? How? Costy and I had no idea. All we knew was that his blue Oldsmobile stopped in front of a garage attached to a house. This was our new abode. The house was a one-floor home with an enormous screened-in porch, part of which my uncle had turned into his private study. There was a master bedroom with a bath in the back, and Costy and I had our own rooms toward the front, with a bathroom between us. The kitchen was much larger than the one in Ithaca, and it opened to an enormous corner of the screen porch. My uncle smoked his pipe in his study/porch, and the absence of a basement led me to believe that perhaps our beatings might come to an end.

Unfortunately, that was not to be. I remember one day when I was vacuuming the living room, and for some reason my uncle was standing in the adjacent dining room, watching me. He began to yell at me, claiming that I was moving the vacuum the wrong way, ruining the carpet. I watched as he then came down the step from the dining room, thinking that he was going to show me how I should vacuum properly. Instead, he approached me, raised his arm, and beat me repeatedly on the neck, the shoulder, and the back.

I realized then that it did not matter where we lived. The only difference was that the Miami house had no basement to which I could escape when Michel was assaulting my brother. I fled instead to my bedroom, where Costy's screams penetrated my ears more effectively; there were no apples to distract me, and no wall to inspire fantasies about the Poe short story. Meanwhile, my aunt Olga still always seemed to disappear during these assaults. I could not help but wonder if she had a sixth sense that told her when her husband would be transformed into a monster.

My high school years were in Miami, and my memory blocks out those years. Did I ride a bus to school? I have no idea. Did I socialize with friends? I have no idea. What stands out most vividly in my mind is that books became my companions. I read volume after volume by Charles Dickens. Perhaps it was the misery in those books that appealed to me. I was not terribly happy in high school. I remember that students had beach parties, especially after graduation. My uncle drove me to the beach, but I simply walked through the sand alone. I could hear some laughter as I walked, endlessly it seemed, lost in my own thoughts.

The high school gave a prize, the Silver Knight Award, to the best language student. I remember my disappointment when I was only the first runner-up. I had studied German and Spanish, and, of course, my French was fluent. In retrospect, I believe that no one took seriously the fact that I knew no English on arrival in America, that it was a foreign language for me.

Olga, meanwhile, had found a church to which she could walk on Sundays. As was her custom, she would place the Sunday roast in the oven so that it could be ready for Sunday dinner, which was typically, as it had been since our arrival in America, in the middle of the day. Costy and I accompanied her to the services, and we were both baptized by being dunked in a tub of water while church members prayed around us. I understood that this was supposed to be a great personal transformation, but I felt nothing. I simply went along. Being hauled from church to church (one Protestant denomination in Ithaca, another one in Miami—based ultimately on walking distance) only estranged me from any true spirituality. As for my Catholic and Eastern Christian upbringing in Lebanon, that seemed farther away than ever. In fact, it was merely hibernating in a forgotten corner of my psyche.

***

What I had to do during high school was earn some real money for college. I had been accepted into Cornell University, where my tuition would be covered since I was officially the daughter of a faculty member, albeit one who had retired. But I needed money to pay for my room in the dorm, for clothing, and other expenses.

I remember my first job vividly. I walked to a cafeteria in a shopping area not far from our house that had posted a wanted ad for a server. I talked to the manager, who had me fill out a form. He discovered that I had had no previous work experience and informed me that he could not hire me precisely for that reason. I was in a state of disbelief. I said to him that it was impossible for me to have job experience if no one hired me. If he did not hire me, how could I ever get a job anywhere? I would have no experience. He looked at me, laughed, and hired me on the spot.

So I got a uniform (all servers wore one) and showed up for work the next day. The work was not exactly challenging. The servers were all women, and I was probably the youngest. My job was to stand behind food platters. As customers picked up a tray, they would move along and request a specific dish, and whoever was standing behind that food choice would take a large spoon, load it with food, and unload it gently onto the customer's plate.

At the end of the dinner shift (which I worked), the servers were in charge of the food cleanup (a dishwasher was responsible for cleaning customers' dishes). The cleaning was fairly simple. If the food was gone, we would simply hand the metal containers to the dishwasher and wipe up the metal counter. If we wanted to eat, we could serve ourselves from the leftovers.

Many were the nights when all the women, including myself, would sit at one table with plates of food and have dinner while gossiping. There were women of all ages, including elderly women. Some of the women were married, some divorced: some had children, some did not, and some were single. Sitting together after standing for hours serving customers was always a relief. No subject was taboo. Sometimes we would even laugh at some of the more peculiar customers. I must confess that I truly enjoyed that job, perhaps most of all because it got me out of my uncle's house, and I was experiencing a completely new world. Our boss was not overly strict, and I loved the stories the women told as we shared food.

***

After working at the cafeteria for a while, I realized that I was not earning a great deal of money. So I decided to add another job. Not far from the cafeteria was a drugstore that featured a soda fountain and served sandwiches and light food at the counter. I applied for a job there, and since I already had a job in the cafeteria, I was offered the soda fountain job immediately.

Working at a soda fountain was completely different from working at a cafeteria, although I was doing both jobs. The soda fountain started early in the day, and I had to learn a lot more than I needed to know in the cafeteria. I had never had a milkshake in my life. So now I not only tasted a milkshake, but I learned to make one on order. I stood behind a long counter, and customers sat directly in front of me on little stools, arms resting on the counter of the soda fountain.

The money I earned went into a bank account in my name and that of my uncle, but in a tutelary arrangement that gave him complete control over the funds. He did not know, however, the exact amount of money I made. True, he knew my salary, but he was unaware of the tips customers sometimes left on the counter. So I took the opportunity to buy myself a small radio with an earphone attachment to listen to when I walked from the house to my jobs.

One day, during my last summer in Miami, I was vacuuming the living room rug as usual. My uncle began to yell that I was doing it wrong as he came toward me. I knew what would follow. He raised his arm. Without thinking, and before his arm could come down on me, I struck him hard on the back of his neck. He stepped back, stunned, and he never hit me again.

Between the two jobs and going to high school, I did not have much time to spend with my brother. His room was directly across mine in the house, but we rarely talked. I do remember that Costy had to work in the yard, pulling weeds. At one point, Michel decided to get a little dog he named "Happy." Happy ran around the house yapping and kept Michel company while he sometimes sat outside and pulled weeds alongside Costy. Happy must not have been very happy because she did not stay with the family long and ran away instead. My uncle walked around the entire neighborhood, asking people if they had seen Happy. Unlike us humans, Happy could escape. I actually felt sorry for my uncle when he lost that dog.

My last weeks in Florida were spent shopping, mostly in used clothing stores. I was ecstatic at the idea of getting out of Miami to attend Cornell. Now, when my uncle began his screaming routines, I barely heard him. I figured that he was serenading me so I would never forget his voice (which I never have). True, I was also being separated from Costy, but at the time, all I could think about was escape and a new life.

I was nervous about going back to Ithaca, lest I be overtaken by those horrific memories from the days we lived there with my uncle. But somehow, when I arrived at Cornell University as an entering freshman, I did not think much about Mitchell Street and the life my brother and I led there. In fact, I never set foot on that street the entire time I was at Cornell. For me, that street was cursed, and nothing but evil could come of my even seeing it.

CHAPTER 18

Cornell

Cornell was a challenging academic environment. When I look back on my education, I can see that other students at Cornell were far better prepared than I was for the coursework. By preference, I took courses in art history and foreign languages. When a requirement came along, like a political science course, I was completely lost. While, to anyone who talked to me, I seemed completely fluent in English, my ability to navigate intellectually demanding English-language materials was not up to the level of my fellow Ivy League students.

Even worse, I had to work to be able to afford school. Many were the mornings when I would watch my dorm roommate awaken nice and spry and head for her classes while I was barely able to get out of bed. I worked in the Willard Straight Hall cafeteria, where most students ate, bussing tables late into the night. What remains with me from that period of my life is the sense of exhaustion with which I awoke most mornings and with which I fell asleep almost every night.

That first year, and to my great surprise, I also began to receive letters from Aunt Najla addressed directly to me at the dorm. I kept those letters for years. Aunt Najla had no idea of our family situation with Michel. I never wrote to tell her or Mama Hana about the physical and emotional abuse my brother and I endured. My memories of Aunt Najla had always been positive. But when I began to receive her letters during my first year at Cornell, I had to readjust my understanding of her. She wrote me in English and not Arabic or French, something that surprised me at first but to which I became accustomed.

At first, I did not think very much about her addressing letters to my Cornell address. But as the letters piled up, I realized that she was working in collusion with my uncle. How else would she have known my dorm address? Her words were often harsh, and I barely recognized the Aunt Najla I knew from my days in Deir el-Amar. Her missives were short and to the point: she understood that I was missing some of my classes, she chastised me for not staying in close contact with my uncle, she repeated over and over that Michel and his family had brought me and Costy to America so we would have the wonderful life we could not have had had we stayed in Lebanon, and so on, and so on. I never wrote back to Aunt Najla. What would have been the point? Besides, I was certain that whatever I wrote, be it about life with Michel or life at Cornell, would have simply made it back to my uncle. I felt more isolated than comforted by these epistles from someone I had trusted and loved as a child.

More dramatic was my fall one gorgeous summer day (I believe it was the summer between my freshman and sophomore years). I was walking from the Olin library with a fellow student worker to have lunch in the Straight. The scene is so alive in my mind that I remember exactly what I was wearing: a lime-green, short-sleeved jersey shirt and a flowered skirt that I bought at a five-and-dime store. With this outfit, I wore flat cotton sandals from the same store. It was a work outfit, perfect for those hot and often humid Ithaca days.

My colleague and I were talking as we walked, and before I knew it, I had fallen in the middle of the street, with cars passing me by. I had inadvertently tripped on the edge of the sidewalk and had a cut on my right leg that stretched from my knee almost to my feet. I was in great pain and could not move. Blood was flowing everywhere. My colleague ran back to the library and called an ambulance.

The next thing I remember was being in a hospital bed, my colleague by my side and my right leg full of stitches. How long was I in the hospital? Did they pump me full of pain killers? The details of that fall pale compared to what I had to do next. Michel held the money I had earned in Miami as well my earnings from Cornell in the Florida account he controlled. I had some money for daily expenses, but a hospital bill required more. There was no way out. I had to call Michel and ask him to pay the hospital bill from my account.

I vividly remember trying to keep his voice away from my ear by holding the phone at a distance. It was a silly action on my part because his screams penetrated my head anyway. I lost count of the number of times he called me "You stupid *sharmouta*." I was actually surprised that he had the energy to say it over and over. I could see him in my mind's eye in the Florida house, pacing back and forth on the screened-in porch as he pushed the words out of his mouth. I let him spew his bile because to stop him would have been like stopping a raging bull. I had fallen, he insisted, because I was wearing high heels (which I wasn't) like a *sharmouta*. I was a *sharmouta* and would end my days in the gutter.

I must have hung up the phone at some point, but that remains a gap in my memory (and Michel did pay the bill). What is not a gap in my memory is the scar still visible on my right leg. What also remains to this day is the far greater emotional scar. Despite my professional success (and despite my husband's denegations), part of me continues to believe that my uncle spoke the truth, that

I will end my days in the gutter. The psychological fallout from a call to Michel was always the same. I would collapse into depression. I would curse my fate. Of course, I did not know then that this fall was just a first greeting from the Charcot-Marie-Tooth muscular dystrophy that would invade my adulthood.

***

When I was not working in the cafeteria, I would go to the music room in the Straight and listen to classical music. The music room was a largely gay hangout, but I did not care. Drowning myself in Mozart or Beethoven was more important to me than being in a room with gay students. Sexual orientation meant nothing to me then, just as it means nothing to me now. It was through the music room that I met Allen, my future husband. At parties, when someone asks how we met, Allen likes to say we were introduced by a bisexual who was interested in both of us and who lost out all around. One day—January 29, 1967, to be exact—while I was bussing tables at the Straight, an acquaintance from the music room waved me over and in the process introduced me to a young man with whom he was having coffee. Our accidental matchmaker was very gracious, allowing us to use his apartment for our first night together.

At Cornell in those days, there were over five male students for every three coeds. We called it the ratio. So it is not surprising that I never lacked for boyfriends. But it took me less than a week to realize that Allen was different. Of course, it did not hurt that I found him irresistibly sexy (and still do). His hair varied from light brown to sandy, depending on its exposure to the sun. His eyes—his eyes were like the sea. I could lose myself in them as they changed from blue to grey. He was tall (over six feet) and trim. His chest was smooth and hairless. He had just turned seventeen, and I had just turned twenty-one. He was a freshman; I was in the middle of my sophomore year.

More important, I soon discovered that Allen was an exceptionally intense young man, both intellectually and emotionally, and exceptionally generous with money and with affection. We shared everything. Every semester, we arranged to have at least one course in common. One of Allen's in-laws once described us as co-dependent—psychobabble for mutually clingy. There have been times (we have been together almost half a century) when this closeness could feel stifling. But for most of my adult life, I have found Allen a strong and steady pillar. I used to kiddingly refer to an ad from the late sixties for women's pants: A Man You Can Lean on—That's Klopman. At the time, my reference was primarily emotional. Now I lean on Allen for physical support as well.

***

My sophomore year at Cornell made me realize that I needed a break from college. Not only were my jobs barely keeping me alive, but at times Allen would pay for my meals when we ate in the Straight cafeteria. I decided to take a leave of absence from Cornell and go to New York City. My hope was to get a job, earn some real money, and then return to Cornell for my junior year.

I headed for New York on a bus and, on arrival, went directly to the YWCA, where I had a small room that became my home for a few weeks. I started looking for a job and was fortunate to get one at a legal firm connected to Columbia University. The woman who interviewed me told me she was impressed that I could type in both English and French. I became part of a secretarial pool with my own station: a chair, a table, and a typewriter. I was surrounded by other women whose job was identical to mine.

A coworker took me aside one day and said she needed to speak to me. We had to wait for the lunch break, and I spent the morning wondering if I had done something wrong. When the time came, my colleague walked me out to the hallway and proceeded to give me a speech. The upshot of her lecture was that I was typing too fast, and the typing pool felt that I was making everyone else look bad. I needed to slow down my work. I was flabbergasted. But I needed the money, and the job was better than that of a waitress, so I made an effort to slow down, though the act of waiting before striking a typewriter key tried my patience. I have always thought of myself as a hard worker, but I must also be an unusually fast one. I have found people telling me to slow down throughout my professional life.

Once I had the job at the legal firm, I looked for a place to live. I ended up sharing a one-bedroom apartment with two other young women who were also working in the city as secretaries. The tiny apartment was quite nice, in a building with a doorman on Fifth Avenue near Fourteenth Street. I loved living in New York. After I got my first check, I went out to buy dresses suitable for a secretary in a New York law firm. The area where we girls lived was full of little boutiques with inexpensive wear for young women like us.

Living and working in a big city like New York was a radical change. During that year, I met Allen's mother, who lived in Queens. A teacher in an elementary school, she invited me to come and speak to her students. One evening, we got high together on some pot given to her by her boyfriend (she was divorced from Allen's father). It was the first time I had ever smoked marijuana. I now realize what I felt in New York that year was a great sense of liberation. I had managed to push the Malti family to the back of my mind. Were they thinking about me? I never even asked myself the question.

***

When I returned to Cornell for my junior year, I was in for a surprise. At the time, the children of Cornell faculty, if they were accepted, received free tuition from the university, something from which all the Malti children had benefited, and which was extended to me since legally I was Michel's adopted daughter. Upon my return to Ithaca, I received a call from the office of the University Provost. His secretary said he wanted to see me and made an appointment. When I arrived, she escorted me to his private suite where he was already hosting a guest: the famous Israeli archeologist, Yigal Yadin. The two were sitting around a circular table, and I was invited to join them. I did not understand what was going on, and the suspense was killing me.

The Provost, who obviously had no problem speaking to me in front of Yigal Yadin, proceeded to explain why I was there. My uncle Michel, aka Dad, had refused to sign the faculty waiver for my tuition, though of course signing would not cost him a cent. I said not a word. I certainly did not have the means to pay Cornell tuition myself.

I was trying to hold back my tears, knowing that my education was coming to an end. I had no reply to the Provost's words. I was tempted to scream at the Provost and ask him why I had to receive the news like this. Why didn't he just write me a letter? Then I could have digested the bad news in complete privacy and gone about living my life working as a secretary. Michel's refusal, though it came as a surprise, did not really shock me. He had no other way to punish me. His beatings had served no purpose. He was quite intelligent and had obviously concluded that using Aunt Najla to force me to bow to him had not worked, either. Not signing the university papers was his only recourse.

The Provost watched me as I sat in silence. Then he turned to me and proceeded to tell me that he had known Michel for many years, that he was familiar with how he always parked his car illegally, flaunting university rules, that he found him an impossible human being, and that he was not at all surprised by his refusal to sign the papers for me to continue my education. All that was running through my head as I listened to the Provost was what Yigal Yadin, sitting quietly in his own chair, could possibly be thinking. Why that should have mattered to me remains a mystery.

Then the Provost, still looking at me, told me that he was going to sign the paper on his own authority, providing me with free tuition. I was stunned. I thanked the Provost profusely for this unexpected gift. I also promised him that I intended to take my studies at Cornell seriously, and that his precious gift would not be wasted. The Provost stood up, and I took that to mean that it was time for me to leave. He assured me that he had faith in me and shook my hand. Yigal Yadin also extended his hand to me as I left the room.

***

So it was that I began my junior year at Cornell with the Provost's generosity and blessings. I felt lucky. I also could not help but think about Michel and his anger when he would hear the news—which he surely would—that I was continuing at Cornell. I confess that I took an almost sadistic pleasure in the thought of his impotent wrath at being bypassed by, of all people, the Provost of the university. I kissed off the bank account in Miami and filled out papers to have myself declared an emancipated minor. I was on my own, and I liked it better that way.

Having spent a year working as a secretary taught me the value of an education. The Provost's generosity was a gift I had not expected. I worked as hard as I could during my junior and senior years at Cornell, and I decided to major in Semitic languages and literatures.

When I first came to Cornell, I assumed I would major in French. My real wish had been to go to Middlebury College and become a French teacher. But the French courses at Cornell were simply not challenging for me. Even the more advanced literature courses were filled with American students still struggling to express themselves in that language, while at this stage of my life, my written French was probably still better than my English. I dabbled for a while with the idea of majoring in German.

Then I noticed that Cornell offered Arabic, and I decided it was time for me to reconnect with that part of my heritage because I had lost all ability to speak or understand my mother tongue. Back in Lebanon, my instruction in literary Arabic had been limited by my young age; by the time I got to college, I could no more decipher a written text than I could express myself in Lebanese dialect. My uncle's de-Arabization program seemed to have achieved its goals.

When I signed up for first-year Arabic in my sophomore year, my only advantage was that I knew the alphabet and could pronounce with ease all those Semitic consonants that are so difficult for a Western tongue. Despite these advantages, I found mastering Arabic—a living, centuries-old classical language—along with its spoken dialects to be a decades-long endeavor.

Arabic was taught in the Department of Semitic Languages and Literatures, along with Hebrew. A major was expected to take three years of a major language, in my case Arabic, and two years of a minor one (in my case, Hebrew). By the time I left Cornell, I was reading, albeit quite imperfectly, the *Qur'an* in Arabic and the *Torah* in Hebrew. I was one of only two students in some of those classes. One day, neither of us showed up to class. In the next class, the professor said something I will never forget. "If neither of you is going to come to class, please let me know, so I don't have to come to campus."

***

Those last two years at Cornell were tumultuous. The Vietnam War was in full swing. The African-American students organized a sit-in at Willard Straight Hall. I spent many a weekend night after parties with Allen in his room at the fraternity house. To pay my Cornell expenses, I again held two jobs, one in the Olin library and the other as a waitress in the restaurant attached to the famous Cornell Statler Hotel School. I would have to wake up early in the morning, put on my waitress uniform, and walk across the dramatic suspension bridge over the gorge from the fraternity house to the Hotel School restaurant. There, I was taught French service, in which the waiter holds a large fork and spoon in the right hand, somewhat like chopsticks, and manipulates them to grab an item of food from a serving dish on the left arm and transfer it elegantly to the diner's plate.

One morning, Dean Rusk, the US Secretary of State, who had spent the night in the Statler Hotel, was seated at a single corner table in my station. I served him his breakfast. His son was a Cornell undergraduate, and his father had come to pay him a visit. When I told my friends that I had waited on Dean Rusk, they all said that I should have thrown the hot coffee in his lap while yelling "Napalm." Obviously, I would never do such a thing, but the suggestion expressed the mood of the times; the Vietnam War was raging.

For a while, I shared an apartment in College Town with another undergraduate. The bedroom was huge, but someone (it could have been my roommate, but I am not certain) had covered an entire wall opposite the bed with a reproduction of Goya's dramatic *The Third of May 1808*. The painting, in which French soldiers execute pathetic Spanish civilians whose blood stains the ground, is a searing indictment of anti-guerilla warfare. Allen and I found it so disturbing that we covered it with one of those enormous patterned Indian bedspreads that were so popular in the 1960s.

One weekend, there was a dressy party at Allen's fraternity, and I happened to be sitting in his room all fancied up, awaiting the festivities. Allen was told he had a female visitor. Neither of us recognized the name, so we both went out to greet this unexpected guest. The scene is so alive in my mind that I relive it as I turn it into words. Allen and I were wearing our party clothes; I was in a cocktail dress and high heels, and he was in a three-piece suit. We walked from his room to the top of the stairs overlooking the fraternity's front door. There was Michel's daughter, Connie. Allen began walking down the steps, not recognizing the visitor, who asked him, "Is that my sister?" He only remembers his confusion at the question, whereas I remember my anger. What the hell was she doing there? How did she know where I was? As soon as she saw me, she turned around and left. Put simply, she was spying on me at Michel's behest, which I considered an act of betrayal after all we had shared.

Summers in Ithaca were a special time for Allen and me. Even though his family home was only a few hours away in New York City, he spent all his college summers in Ithaca with me. I held a variety of jobs. Summers were the time for me to work even more hours: up to sixty a week.

One job (which I also held during the year) was at Johnny's Big Red Grill in College Town, near the campus. It was the kind of place that is a little uptown for students but can appeal to some townies or to students whose parents were paying. We served Italian-American food and had a full bar. One regular customer always ordered a whole fish and ate only the skin, leaving the flesh behind. Another customer, an elderly gentleman, had a fixed routine: upon his arrival, he would be served a Manhattan, and five minutes later, a second.

At Johnny's, I learned the seamier side of the restaurant business. One day, when I was in the kitchen, I saw a roach fall from the ceiling into a large soup pot. I tried to retrieve it with a ladle, but the insect was nowhere to be found, having blended into the contents. I turned to the cook and asked what we were to do. His answer stunned me: Serve the soup anyway. No one would be able to distinguish the roach from the vegetables.

Allen also held a variety of summer jobs. The most colorful was that of field hand on the experimental farms run by the Cornell College of Agriculture. He would return home hot and sweaty and immediately take a shower. One of the most beautiful times on the Cornell campus was summer break, when most students had gone and an almost languorous atmosphere descended on Cornell's green hills, now-empty buildings, and rushing streams.

In my senior year, I applied to graduate schools. I was accepted at the University of Pennsylvania. When we two students showed up to Arabic class in the spring semester, the professor asked what we were doing next. My colleague was going to graduate school—Berkeley, I believe. When the professor asked me, I said Penn. He seemed not to recognize the name and said, "What is that?"

I answered "the University of Pennsylvania."

He replied: "You are going to the University of Pennsylvania?"

"Yes," I said.

He was clearly in shock, though he attempted to hide it. "Good for you," he forced himself to say. Penn was one of the top schools in the field of Middle Eastern studies, and clearly this professor did not think me worthy of such an honor. When I had earlier made inquiries about graduate school, he had told me I should become a librarian.

Years later, I was invited to Harvard for a lecture, and my undergraduate professor was teaching in the Boston area. He called me, after having received the notice about the lecture, and asked me to have a cup of coffee with him—a cup that lasted a couple of hours. It became clear to me while we shared those cups of coffee that he had completely forgotten the earlier episode.

***

Students we knew, who were graduating, were being drafted for the war in Vietnam. Fighting in that war was not something Allen was prepared to do. But to escape conscription (since his lottery number was too low), he needed a medical excuse. Simple: he went to New York, where he visited the psychoanalyst he saw as a child. Not only did she not provide a letter, but she was obviously congratulating herself on what a mature, well-adjusted (i.e., sane) young man this once-neurotic boy had become. With a psychiatrist on the Cornell campus, Allen got the Catch-22 answer: sure, fear of the draft could give anyone an anxiety neurosis.

Allen figured out he would have to do this on his own. He arranged to have his physical at the Syracuse induction center, which was reputed to be less severe than the one in New York City to which he had been assigned. Once there, he retreated mentally into his childhood psychological misery and avoided all eye contact, especially with the young, attractive female psychiatrist who interviewed all the potential psych cases. It worked. He was free, and I was greatly relieved.

CHAPTER 19

Penn

All too soon, that last summer in Ithaca was ending, and both Allen and I were heading to graduate school: he to UCLA, and I to the University of Pennsylvania. I rented a tiny studio apartment in Philadelphia from which I could walk to the university. I also needed a job to support myself and my graduate studies, since I had received no fellowship from Penn.

I signed up to be a substitute teacher in Philadelphia. I did not need teaching experience. The bachelor's degree from Cornell University was sufficient. That meant I would be called up early in the morning when I was needed at a specific school. I was always prepared with my black outfit: a pair of black pants with a black shirt and, when needed, a black coat and boots.

My teaching assignments were always in the ghetto. I would arrive at the school, report to the appropriate office, and be told to which room I should head. Class plans were normally available. If they were not, I could improvise. I never shied away from the job because I found the students not only very interesting but also very eager to learn. I always told them I came from Lebanon, and their intellectual curiosity was insatiable. I was different from their other teachers, and they enjoyed the change.

***

My substitute teaching was possible because I had signed up, as almost all graduate students in Middle Eastern studies had, for two Arabic seminars taught back to back in one afternoon by the greatest name in that field at the University of Pennsylvania: S. D. Goitein. This was his last year of teaching at Penn, after which he was heading to the Princeton Institute for Advanced Study, where he could continue his research without teaching.

I was extremely fortunate because Goitein was more than just a groundbreaking scholar responsible for the analysis of the famous Geniza documents. The Cairo

Geniza was a storage room for documents written in Arabic by the then-flourishing Jewish community of Cairo. Professor Goitein was also the most amazing and generous teacher I met in all my studies.

That year, one seminar was devoted to a work by the famous mystic, al-Qushayri, and the other to a philosophical treatise by al-Muskawayhi. We graduate students came in the first day equipped with the books by al-Qushayri and al-Muskawayhi, and Goitein began by calling on each of us to read and translate. I was a bit lost at first because my undergraduate training in Arabic left a lot to be desired. The students in the seminars spanned the range from first-year graduate students like myself to students already writing their theses, because this was the last chance to study with this star professor at Penn. We students would study together regardless of our ability, which I found unusual but very rewarding.

Goitein's generosity extended beyond the classroom. Since he was teaching two seminars back to back, he would take a break in the middle. Each week he would invite one student to accompany him to the university cafeteria during that break. When it was my turn in the first semester, Professor Goitein marched to the cafeteria at such a clip that I could barely keep up. Then he insisted that I order something. I chose a piece of apple pie. He ordered coffee and insisted that I order something to drink with the pie. I, too, ordered coffee. He then paid for both of us. I dared say nothing but "Thank you so much, Professor Goitein." He waved his hand as if to say "Stop this silliness," and then picked an empty table and sat across from me.

Then the interrogation began. Where was I from? Why was my Arabic accent so good? He was gracious enough not to speak of my knowledge of Arabic. Then he delved into my personal life: Where was I from? Lebanon. Where was my family? My father had died; I was adopted by my uncle, from whom I was estranged. Was I married? No. Did I have a boyfriend? Yes. Where was he? In graduate school at UCLA. What was he studying? French history.

After he gathered all this information, he asked me if I had a fellowship, and I explained to him that I was substitute teaching in the Philadelphia school system. We talked and talked until Prof. Goitein declared that it was time to return to the seminar. Moving at his same quick pace with me struggling to keep up, we were back in the seminar room at the same time as all the other students. Goitein took an interest in all his students. He wanted all of us to succeed personally and professionally. He never quite said it in those words, but it was obvious to anyone who watched him interact with us.

***

I lost a tremendous amount of weight while I was in Philadelphia. I ate no regular meals and was not about to cook for myself in that studio apartment. When I arrived on campus early in the morning on the days I was not substitute teaching, I would grab a Cadbury bar (I had eaten those as a child) and a cup of coffee from a stand, and head for the library. One very rainy morning, I was holding the coffee in one hand and trying to close my wallet with the other. I had shoved the Cadbury bar in my coat. While closing my wallet, a small black and white photo of my father slipped out and fell into the river of water running down the street. Eventually, that water found its way into the sewer. I was in a panic. I tried to put everything down and grab the photo, but it was raining hard, and the water was moving incredibly fast. I bent down and put my hand in the cold water, but the sewer had already swallowed my father's tiny picture. I was devastated. How could I have been so stupid? I decided not to go to the library that day but instead returned to my tiny apartment. Losing the picture was like losing a part of myself.

However, I could not grieve for long. I had to get back to my studies. As the fall semester progressed, most of the graduate students applied to Princeton to finish their studies with Goitein. I decided to apply to UCLA because Allen was already there. Goitein wrote me a recommendation letter, and I was accepted at UCLA.

CHAPTER 20

Los Angeles and Paris

That June (1971), Allen and I were married. The ceremony was performed by a judge of the New York State Supreme Court in that iconic New York County Supreme Court building that is featured in all the episodes of *Law & Order*. The judge was an acquaintance of Allen's grandfather, who hosted a reception for us in his Sutton Place apartment, with its glorious views of the East River. It was a small affair–just Allen's mother, his brother, his maternal grandparents (whose apartment we were in), and his maternal aunt, the feminist author who wrote under the name Elisabeth Fischer. A Lebanese restaurant delivered food, and Allen's grandfather bought a case of New York State champagne. Like mine, Allen's parents were divorced, and his mother and father were not on speaking terms. We visited Allen's father and his new wife shortly after the wedding. No member of my family was present at the ceremonies.

I did not feel the absence of my family as a lack. It was more like a liberation. I would not have minded seeing Costy, but as far as I knew he was still living with my uncle. I felt obscurely then, and am even more convinced now, that a complete break with Michel's family was a condition of my psychological survival. Looking back on my life, I have also become aware that I have an unusual ability to walk away from relationships with family or with colleagues.

***

Allen and I went off to California. UCLA boasted a federally funded Center for Middle Eastern Studies. The department of Near Eastern Languages, where I landed, benefited greatly from the presence of the center. Upon my arrival, I began taking courses with the professor who would eventually become my graduate advisor, Seeger Bonebakker. Professor Bonebakker told me that I should replace Hebrew with Persian as my minor language, to which I later added Ottoman Turkish. Compared to Penn, the graduate students at UCLA were less than dazzling. No one was ever prepared for the classes, and I quickly rose to the top of the heap through the extraordinary device of always doing my homework.

Bonebakker did have a more advanced class, a seminar in medieval Arabic poetry. I asked if I could join it.

"Oh, no, Fedva, he answered" (the Arabic "w" becoming a "v" in his Dutch accent), "this is an advanced seminar with only one student from Germany who is writing his dissertation."

I could, however, Bonebakker added, sit in on the class if I promised to stay silent. The seminar limped along, since the other student, Hartmut, was in the midst of writing his dissertation, and the last thing on his mind was preparing for the class. Eventually, Bonebakker was obliged to ask me if I would take a stab at the material. From then on, I did all the translating.

A few weeks into the course, Bonebakker approached me sheepishly with a request. It seems the university administration was upset because he was teaching a course with no enrolled students, since Hartmut had not formally signed up. Would I be willing to enroll?

"Of course," I said.

A few years ago, when I was invited to give a lecture in Zurich, Hartmut, who in the meantime had built himself a distinguished career as a prize-winning translator, was gracious enough to come down from Bern after all these years. He and I spent an amusing several hours at the reception and dinner, reminiscing about Bonebakker and the good old days.

One bright spot: the Center at UCLA invited a prominent scholar, the head of the Dominican Institute in Cairo, Father Anawati, as a visiting professor. I took two classes with Father Anawati, in both of which I was the only student. We read Islamic theology, especially the famous medieval scholar, al-Ghazali. Father Anawati closed his eyes while I read aloud and translated. Once, thinking him asleep, I stopped cold in mid-sentence. He immediately opened his sparkling eyes to ask me why I had stopped. Father Anawati always had chocolate with him to reward good students. "What is a Father without chocolate?" he liked to say. Not to brag, but I consumed a lot of chocolate under Father Anawati's tutelage.

***

Allen, meanwhile, received a Fulbright to go to Paris for his thesis research (on the French politician, Georges Valois). I had also received a fellowship from UCLA (in previous years I had been a teaching assistant in Arabic), and we went to France. We rented an adorable one-bedroom apartment in the seventh arrondissement (district), on a small street, the Rue de Bourgogne.

Our apartment had a kitchen that, though tiny, had all the essentials. Allen was anxious to practice his culinary skills. We both loved French food, but we obviously could not afford to treat ourselves to expensive restaurants. The Rue de Bourgogne, despite being a small street, had everything: a pharmacy, a butcher, a fruit-and-vegetable store, a bakery, a deli (what the French call a *charcuterie*), a *crémerie* (cheese and dairy shop), cafes, and restaurants, one of which was a Chinese restaurant where we dined when we were feeling extravagant.

All the merchants knew Allen after a few weeks. We had purchased a set of French cookbooks, including a series called *La cuisine des mois* that was specialized by months. Allen decided he wanted to cook wild boar (*sanglier*), since that was in season. So he ordered a leg of *marcassin*, an adolescent boar. No problem, the butcher assured him. Allen headed for the store the day the boar was due to arrive. The butcher, dressed like all Paris butchers in a white outfit, greeted Allen and went to the back to get the meat. He came out with a long leg covered in a thick orange pelt. When Allen saw that, he asked the butcher if he was going to remove the furry outside of the animal. The butcher laughed and explained to the American facing him that he was simply showing him the leg so he could see it was the genuine article. The concierge heard about this, of course, and also had a good laugh.

***

That winter I found myself in Paris with a cold and a severe sore threat. I asked Allen to go to the pharmacy on the corner and speak to the pharmacist. In France, pharmacists act like para-physicians. They ask you about your condition and then prescribe whatever medicine they are able to provide.

"Please get me some Pastilles Valda," I asked my husband.

"Pastilles Valda?"

He had never heard of them. I simply urged him to ask the pharmacist for them. He returned fairly quickly with a pharmacy bag full of goodies. Ignoring all the medicines, I grabbed the Pastilles Valda. Instantly, I became that little girl with short, curly hair, dressed in a dark navy boarding-school uniform, holding a plastic round item identical to the one I had between my hands in Paris: a see-through plastic with some tape surrounding the container and attaching it to its cover.

I held the precious case and dared not move. Nor did I open it, lest I break some kind of spell. I looked at it as though it could bring the past to life, as though it could transport me back to my childhood. Through their see-through protective covering, the little "pastilles" greeted me, in the shape of a small pyramid and bright green in color, each one surrounded by sugar crystals. I pulled the tape and separated the small top from the bottom of the plastic jar. The Pastilles Valda had the identical delicious smell they had when I was a child.

Euphoria enveloped me. I held the item in my left hand and began to pull out a Pastille Valda with the thumb and the forefinger of my right hand. The tips of my fingers were swimming in sugar, but they managed to grab one of the drops, sugar and all, and gently place it on my tongue. Semiconsciously, I licked the sugar off my fingers. The green drop took over my mouth: a complicated taste in which mint dominated. The drop stuck to my tongue, and slowly began to melt. I felt it getting smaller. As soon as I suspected that that drop was about to disappear, I softly slipped another in my mouth. I consumed the Pastilles Valda in Paris as I had in boarding school. Somehow I could never have enough of them. They were a security blanket, assuring me I had not imagined the past that too often seemed like a creation of my imagination, a fantasy world that never existed.

***

We had a good friend in Paris, Danielle, whom we had known since our Cornell days. She was a schoolteacher and lived with her parents. Once we moved into our apartment on the Rue de Bourgogne, Danielle would drop by unannounced, sometimes spending the night on our living room couch. She would often come in carrying a chocolate bar and ask if we had a baguette. We always had baguettes. She would put the chocolate inside the bread and munch on it. This was not strange to me at all. Growing up in Lebanon, we girls in boarding school ate our chocolate exactly the same way.

By then, 1973, Danielle had a boyfriend who called himself a *docteur ès putes* (doctor of whores). His degree was in mathematics, and he taught at one of the branches of the University of Paris. One night every week, he would drive to the Bois de Boulogne to have sex with a *travelo* (transvestite or transsexual) prostitute. One night, he took us on a guided tour of these erotic woods. Danielle seemed quite accepting of this practice. As she put it, once in a while he just needed to ejaculate "*dans le vide*" (into emptiness), exhibiting French *mores*. Danielle and her friend died a few years later in a head-on collision on a dark Moroccan highway.

***

One day, Allen had an appointment with the famous French historian, Philippe Ariès. He was running late and rushed out of the apartment, heading for the Metro. The Rue de Bourgogne was a narrow one-way street, which was part of what contributed to its charm. But that also meant that cars parked on the sidewalk, and navigating the street on foot could be a challenge. Allen, running to the Metro, ended up running instead into a car parked on the sidewalk. He fell and hit his head on a concrete abutment. Bleeding profusely, he got up and walked to our building, where the concierge spotted him. She ran up calling "Madame, Madame," while he slowly climbed the stairs. As he lay down and we tried to stop the bleeding with towels, the concierge fetched a physician who lived in the building and called an ambulance. The ambulance arrived, and the medics put Allen on a stretcher. I was beside myself. The medics agreed that I could go with him, along with the doctor who accompanied us, in the ambulance as they took him to the Hôpital Laënnec.

The Hôpital Laënnec? I was already feeling overwhelmed. Add to that the name of the hospital, and I confess I no longer knew where my mind had gone. The Hôpital Laënnec was where my father had worked when he completed his medical studies in Paris. All sorts of emotions invaded me. Was Allen's accident one of those predestined events meant to merge my past life with my present one?

Once we arrived at the hospital, Allen was taken in hand by the physicians, and I was asked to leave. Yes, they reassured me, I could come and visit him, but not today. I should call tomorrow, and they would give me a progress report and tell me when I could see him. I have no memory of how I returned to our apartment.

Allen's wound was dramatic, necessitating a row of stitches, but there was no internal damage. He improved rapidly, and I was able to visit him in the hospital. I was not surprised when he spoke of the unusually high quality of the food. I remember him specifically commenting on eating whole artichokes, served with a mustard sauce. Obviously, he had to pull the artichoke leaves and dip them in the sauce, but that did not seem to be a problem. I knew then that he was returning to his old self and would be home soon. After a few days in the hospital, Allen came home to finish his recuperation. I fixed him ground horse meat from the neighborhood Boucher Chevaline (horse butcher) because of its iron content, which is higher even than that of beef, and Allen loved the slightly gamey flavor.

***

Once Allen had fully recovered, we went back to our routines. Every morning, we would make our way to the Bibliothèque Nationale. Allen would head to the right, where he worked in the enormous main reading room, and I would climb a set of stairs on the left to a separate section, the Oriental room, which held Arabic, Hebrew, Chinese, Japanese, and other Oriental manuscripts.

I had a regular seat in the Oriental room. One day I realized that sitting next to me was Georges Vajda, the prominent scholar who worked on Near Eastern manuscripts. Vajda was also the head of a section at the Centre National de la Recherche Scientifique, known as the CNRS. The CNRS covers different branches of the sciences (including the hard sciences), politics, languages, and so on. Vajda was the head of a team at the IRHT, the Institut de Recherche et d'Histoire des Textes, that concentrated on the computerization of medieval Arabic biographical dictionaries (a technology that was then in its infancy).

Vajda invited me to join his team, and I was appointed as a *chercheur* (researcher) at the CNRS. I had never worked on biographical dictionaries, a fascinating area that had not been included in my studies at UCLA. I loved reading the medieval biographies. It was almost like reading the gossip of a bunch of scholars from centuries past. In addition, this evolved into a salaried position, which permitted us to spend another entire year in Paris.

Paris was where I began my publishing career. I published two articles, both in prominent international journals, *Arabica* and the *Journal Asiatique*. The latter was the journal of the Société Asiatique to which I was admitted under the patronage of Georges Vajda. As the prolific Byzantinist, Speros Vryonis, said to me when I returned to California, I had been bitten by the bug. That bug was the bug of publishing. But it was not just me. I was associated with a group of scholars for whom publishing was not something extraordinary. The French system did not possess the same demarcation between graduate students (who were studying to become scholars) and professors (who were expected to publish scientific research). It was not apprentices versus masters. We were all involved in the pursuit and dissemination of new knowledge.

Years, books, and over a hundred articles later, I understand that my fundamental passion is writing. Starting in high school and continuing in college, I had kept a diary (first in French and then in English). I now understand that scholarly publishing was the vehicle that permitted me to express my largely unconscious drive to write. Publishing my own prose (for a specialist in a foreign literature, I did relatively little translation) was the part of my university career I liked best.

Living in Paris for such a long period made France a second home for us. For me, it was also a vital intellectual influence. I had come to Paris to study Medieval Arabic prose anecdotes by reading works in manuscript at the Bibliothèque Nationale, but I had no sense of what to do with what I was reading. Browsing in the giant bookstores of the Boulevard Saint-Michel, I came across that group of French thinkers—linguists, anthropologists, and literary critics—usually called structuralists. They opened a new world to me, one I was able to exploit not only in my dissertation but in my later work as well.

France also brought me back to the Catholic Church. That first Christmas in Paris, I told Allen I wanted to attend Midnight Mass in Notre Dame Cathedral. It was packed (Allen bumped into an enormous candle, spilling wax on my coat). The ceremony was as impressive as one would expect. I was stirred to hear the Christmas carols I knew from my childhood (*Il est né le Divin Enfant*). I knew then that I could drop in on a Catholic Church anywhere I was in Europe. A few years later, I started visiting Saint Patrick's when we were in New York. Despite loving to attend high masses, I have always kept the institution of the Church at arm's length. I have never joined a parish at any of the places we have lived.

CHAPTER 21

Rites of Passage

When we returned to California in 1975, we both continued working on our dissertations, mine on Medieval Arabic literature and Allen's on modern French history. One day, I had a meeting with a member of my dissertation committee, with whom I had studied comparative literature. He was extremely knowledgeable about all the new developments in literary theory (including the French structuralists). I was excited by these developments and was grateful to Ross Shideler for being such a generous mentor.

But my meeting with Ross was not all positive. He revealed to me that he had recently had a chat with my dissertation advisor, Prof. Bonebakker. Bonebakker confessed to Ross that he did not understand what I was doing in my dissertation. Ross reassured him that my work was on the cutting edge of the field, that what I was writing made complete sense to him, and that Bonebakker should not worry about it.

While I was writing my dissertation, Bonebakker insisted that he had to read what I was writing immediately. At the time, I was writing in notebooks that I would type later. He insisted on having the notebooks full of my handwriting. Personally, I found this a bit obsessive, but I complied with his wishes. He had trouble reading my handwriting and, after reading two or three notebooks, gave up and said he would wait to read the typed text.

Meeting with Bonebakker in his office, up a set of steep stairs, was always troublesome. At times, as I was leaving those meetings, I would feel anxious and lose my balance on the stairs. I never actually fell, but I could feel the tension in my body.

I began applying for jobs. Nothing. I was getting nowhere. I spoke to a friend, who was completing her dissertation in American history. Our friend laughed and asked me if I had seen what was in my employment dossier. Of course not, I told her; that was confidential. She laughed and told me I was a fool. Graduate students looking for a job, she was quick to reveal, had their dossier sent to a friend and could then see what kinds of letters lurked inside. She offered me her address, so I could have my dossier sent to her. I hesitated. What if the office where these materials were kept realized that I had requested that my dossier be sent to a local address? Allen encouraged me to do what our friend suggested, which I did.

When the dossier arrived in our friend's mailbox, she handed it right over to me. I was extremely nervous, and as soon as we got home, I asked Allen to open it and read the letters. Suddenly, I could tell by the look on his face that he was reading a poison-pen letter. As I suspected, Bonebakker had written a negative letter that was blocking me everywhere. Fortunately, I had taken to going to professional meetings where I had met some highly placed scholars. Three scholars, none of whom served on my doctoral committee, became my mentors and recommenders: Muhsin Mahdi, the Jewett professor of Arabic at Harvard, who held the most important Arabic chair in the country; George Makdisi, who had replaced Goitein at Penn after my departure and shared my Lebanese-Christian origins; and finally Speros Vryonis, the director of the Von Grunebaum Middle East Center at UCLA, who also became a lifelong supporter and friend. A few years later, Mohammed Arkoun, Professor of Islamic Philosophy at the Sorbonne, joined the group. With backers like these, my employment fortunes changed. In a young scholar's life, the dissertation advisor (usually a male) acts as a kind of surrogate father. Making my career without my dissertation advisor (I never asked Bonebakker for anything again) made me a kind of academic orphan. I adapted to this situation much as I had adapted to my biological and legal orphanhood.

When I saw an advertisement for a lectureship in Arabic at San Diego State, I begged my contacts to write letters of recommendation. Surprise of surprises, I got the job. Allen and I were both ecstatic because this represented real money and not simply a fellowship.

We rented an adorable little house on a hillside in San Diego. I loved that house because of its colors. Walking into the living room was like walking into a rainbow. The wall-to-wall carpet was made up of rug pieces of different bright colors sewn together. The patching was invisible. Gazing at the floor was like immersing yourself in a painting. I imagined while we lived there that this must have been what Joseph's coat of many colors looked like.

It was 1977, the year I would receive my PhD and begin my professional career at the age of thirty-one. I received a tenure-track appointment at the University of Virginia for the following year. The move to the East coast was fast approaching, as was the end of my interim year of teaching in San Diego.

Ever since Cornell, I had become increasingly aware that I had a tendency to limp, especially at the end of a long day. More recently, descending the steep stairs from Bonebakker's office, I often felt as if I were going to fall, though I attributed this to nervousness. Every time I crossed an important barrier, I felt that my life was beginning anew. I had always tried to bury the past, to abandon it like a corpse that would remain safely in its hole in the ground. Crossing the country to a new position was definitely crossing a boundary. I was excited at the possibility that I might be able to fix my walk at the same time I received my PhD. We had some friends in San Diego, Tom and Doris, a physician and his wife who were close friends of Allen's brother, Peter, also a physician. I asked Tom about my limp, and he mentioned that there was a gait clinic at the San Diego Hospital. They should be able to figure out the cause of my limp. Who knows, maybe one of my legs was shorter than the other.

Soon, I found myself, together with Allen, in the waiting room of a neurologist at the hospital. The only available seats were next to an elderly woman. No one spoke, as if words might break a fragility born of isolation, of vulnerability. Most eyes faced down. Like everyone else, I spent my time avoiding other people's gazes. This was before medical waiting rooms numbed their patients' minds with endless television.

Glancing down, I noticed my female neighbor's feet trying to hide beneath the thin leather straps of her open sandals. I was struck by the skin on her toes. It was shriveled, reminding me of uncooked chicken skin. I could see no muscles, and the pores stood out as they do on chicken skin. The sight frightened me, as if this woman had the feet of an animal.

I could not see my own feet, since I was wearing a pair of multicolored ankle-high shoes purchased in Paris. Did my feet look like that? If I had to guess, I would have said no. I polished my toenails when I wore sandals, especially in California, a place destined for such self-indulgence, and had never noticed anything like what was staring at me in the neurologist's office. The vision of the chicken skin embedded itself in my brain. No, I said to myself, my skin would never look like that.

My turn finally came. I limped into the imposing examination room, Allen by my side. At last, the neurologist entered. He was tall and thin, with a kindly face. He was friendly and conducted a full examination of my reflexes, touching my feet and toes and asking me to move them. Not only could I not do so, but I had not even been aware that I could not. The neurologist probed some more and finally concluded:

"I think you have muscular dystrophy. I could, of course, be wrong. But we need to take more tests, and if it is MD, we need to find the cause."

Muscular dystrophy. These two words sent my head reeling. I read my own terror in Allen's sudden pallor. The neurologist was quick to speak, attempting to reassure us both. "Muscular Dystrophy doesn't have to mean Duchenne's syndrome. There are many forms of dystrophy, each caused by something different."

That was little comfort—like hearing that there are many forms of cancer, each caused by something different. I could not forget that vision of the chicken skin.

"Will my skin shrivel and look like chicken skin?" I asked the physician.

"Chicken skin?" he answered with surprise in his voice.

He clearly had no idea what had prompted my question.

"No. Your skin will look perfectly normal."

I was reassured. After all, if the neurologist could predict the future, why should I argue with him? Now, I look at my hands and recognize the chicken skin I had seen on that woman's feet in San Diego. It is there on my own hands, between the fingers, especially between the thumb and index finger. Now I understand its cause. The atrophied muscles leave the skin flabby, without underlying support, looking like the skin of a dead chicken. It is on my feet, arms, and legs as well. But my hands stare at me almost every minute of the day, reminding me of that woman so long ago who probably was also reassured by her neurologist, as I had been, that her skin would remain perfectly normal.

There are blessings to being young. One wants to believe the best, that the world can be conquered, and that one's body can also be conquered. So when the neurologist suggested we start with a blood test, both Allen and I agreed. That was the bottom of the ladder. Some dystrophies could be caused by a vitamin B deficiency.

"What would that mean?" I asked.

"You would need to come to the hospital once a week and receive injections of vitamin B."

"Oh, my God," I gasped. "That's awful." The neurologist admitted that this was not a pleasant prospect but suggested we wait and see what the blood results showed.

It was a horrible week, and all I could think of were those shots. I wished that I had never taken Tom's advice and exposed my body to the world of medicine. We returned to the hospital and met with the same neurologist. "It's not vitamin B deficiency," he informed us. I breathed a sigh of relief.

Little did I know that once I placed my foot on the first step of that medical ladder, I was doomed to keep climbing toward one possibility after another. With each new diagnostic guess, we moved up the medical rungs to more complicated and more serious conditions. How I longed for that first speculation, which had created such shudders, of vitamin B. Alas, the neurologist's other conjectures went the way of that vitamin. Blissfully, I have forgotten them all.

We were back where we began. As a last resort, the neurologist suggested I undergo an EMG, an electromyogram, explaining the procedure to us. Needles would be placed in different sections of my arms, legs, feet, and hands. An electric current would be activated through the needle. The purpose was to demonstrate the ability of my nerves to transmit orders to my muscles so that the latter would do what they were meant to do.

Allen and I arrived at the hospital early in the morning, and I was guided to the bowels of the building, where the EMG would be performed. I was alone and shaking with fright. "Caution: Radiation" signs marked the walls. Once I undressed, put on a hospital gown, and lay on the table, it was too late to run away. I was told the EMG would cause discomfort. I did not understand the euphemisms of the medical profession. The word *discomfort* should be translated into everyday parlance as severe pain. (Mild discomfort means pain.)

Suddenly, the neurologist was standing by my side, surrounded by other males clad in white. My condition was so rare. Would I mind if others observed the procedure? I raised my head. Did I have a choice? I was a guinea pig, a medical object. Lying there naked with only my hospital robe tied loosely around my body already made me feel vulnerable. But then to be asked to be the circus freak whose performance would have an audience left me speechless. The neurologist was looking at my face, and I was certain he could see my discomfort. I felt I had no choice in the matter.

When the neurologist had explained the procedure, it had all sounded so innocent. The staff started planting the needles in my body: my arms, my legs. When it was time, a hand would appear as if from nowhere and move the needle around the area where it was planted while the electric current was transmitted through the needle to my body.

It was time for the show to begin. The nurse turned my body around so that I faced the wall. My head rested on a pillow. Then I felt her hand on my back, beginning to untie the robe one knot at a time. The neurologist began inserting needles in my leg and thigh muscles. As a needle penetrated my flesh, he would move it around. I told myself he was involved in performance art. As the needle moved, I assumed it was leaving a track. But the needles were only the beginning. We would soon move to the nerves. The nerves received electric shocks to activate them so their performance could be judged. I imagined a ballet taking place in my body as the muscles and nerves began their induced dance.

How long did this dance last? I have no idea. I was creating scenarios of waltzes in my brain to distract myself from the pain. I imagined the muscles as ladies being led on the dance floor by the nerves. But this was not a normal choreography. This was an artificially created ballet in which muscles and nerves had to be pushed into dancing. As I attempted to distract myself with these silly ideas, the pain continued, providing the background scenery for this strange performance.

Like the director of an orchestra, the neurologist signaled the nurse, who would twist the needle and push it in further as the machine behind him spat out the results on paper. The words of the neurologist to his colleagues flowed continuously, just like the electric current.

Discomfort? A lovely term, indeed. I had never felt such intense pain. When the needles were rotated in my thighs, I could not help but sob. I pressed my face against the cold hospital wall as the warm tears wet my skin. I cried for the remainder of the procedure. Once the torture was over, the males exited, leaving me alone with the nurse. I felt ashamed, weak. The nurse reassured me: even men cry during this ordeal. Was that supposed to be comforting?

I put on my clothing and was directed out of the room to the area where Allen was waiting. The look on his face betrayed a host of emotions. The nurse had already informed me that we would not have the results of the EMG until they had been read by the appropriate physicians.

We got into the car and began the drive home. I could barely see the road because of the tears blocking my vision. Allen suggested that we drive to a favorite spot on the coast. I nodded. One could walk down to the rocks close to the ocean where the waves crashed on the enormous stones with loud whooshes. It was an idyllic space. Sunsets over the Pacific Ocean were so spectacular that they could bring tears to your eyes. How long did we sit watching the waves splash up against the rocks? I do not remember. What I remember is Allen looking at me with worry in his eyes. We held hands, and he tried to dry the tears rolling down my face. Neither of us said a word. There are times and places in life where words do not belong.

As it began to get dark, Allen stood up and, his hand still in mine, helped me to stand. We hugged each other and headed for the car. We heard nothing but the sound of the waves bidding us goodbye. We drove home without uttering a word. I parked the car, Allen opened the door of our little house, and Joseph's coat of many colors silently welcomed us home.

***

The neurologist had been right. I had muscular dystrophy. He guessed that it was most likely a form of dystrophy called Charcot-Marie-Tooth disease, known by its initials as CMT. CMT was a peripheral neuropathy that was not only hereditary but also degenerative; that is, it would get worse as I got older. I do not believe I heard a word the neurologist said. I was nostalgically yearning for that vitamin B deficiency and its cousins, whose diagnoses were now history. The neurologist's voice broke through my reflections.

"Does anyone in your family have this disease?" he asked.

"I don't know," I heard myself replying.

"Family history is very important in these diagnoses." He was droning on. "In fact, family history could be the most important factor here."

His words flew by me like sparrows fleeing a hawk. How could I explain to him that my family was nonexistent? That my mother had long ago disappeared from my life? That the corpse of my father, buried halfway around the globe, had likely decomposed by now? That I had long ago lost track of my aunt Najla and did not know if she was dead or alive? That I was not on speaking terms with my uncle or his family? How could I explain to him that in the Middle East, such things are a source of shame, and no one speaks of them? How could I explain to him that a medical history was an absurdity in a culture in which I did not even know when I was born?

For lack of what to say, I assured the neurologist that I would look into the matter and get back to him with an answer. He requested that I make another appointment to see him. "It's very important," his voice was going on, "for us to determine the final diagnosis. We can't do that without knowing if anyone else in your family has the condition."

Chapter 22

Constantine

How much time did we spend with the neurologist? I have no idea. But of one thing I was sure: we eventually left the hospital and returned to our colorful carpet. I felt like a stranger in an even stranger body. I was losing track of who I was. I did not recognize this body that had its own genetic plans and was forcing me to adapt to them.

Allen, always the level-headed one in the family, decided that we should call my brother Constantine, with whom I had lost touch. I had been so eager to get away from Michel and his family that I effectively left Constantine as well. Since he was still living with my uncle at the time, he was, in my mind, part of the world from which I had fled. But, as Allen was quick to point out, he was my only full-blood relative, and if we could speak to him, we might learn something. I told Allen that there was no way I was calling my uncle, and that he would have to make the call himself. I warned him Michel might just hang up on him.

The scene is as alive for me today as it was in San Diego almost four decades ago. Allen picked up the phone and dialed the number in Miami. I stood by his side, hearing only his part of the conversation.

"May I speak to Constantine Malti, please?"

[...]

"Oh, he's not there? Do you know how I can reach him?"

[...]

"Yes, that would be very nice. Thank you."

I then saw Allen reach for a pen and scribble down a number.

"Thank you very much. Goodbye."

"Who was on the phone?" I asked.

"A woman."

"It must have been my aunt Olga," I concluded. "Michel would have cursed you and hung up the phone."

I had not seen Constantine for more than a decade. The idea of calling him to ask about a hereditary condition was not one I relished. Allen was pushing me, telling me I would have to do this sooner or later. I finally dialed the number.

"Operator's room," a voice answered.

"May I speak to Constantine Malti, please?"

"He's not here at the moment. Would you like to leave a message?"

"Yes, please. Could you ask him to call his sister at the following number?"

"Sure."

"Thank you very much."

"You're welcome."

Click.

Allen and I dissected every word of that short conversation. We wondered what kind of operator he might be. Was he working for a police department? A detective agency? A hospital? Constantine finally called. He expressed his surprise and pleasure at hearing from us.

I knew the next part would be unbearable. For both of us.

"How are your legs?" I asked.

"I don't want to talk about it," he replied angrily.

"Come on," I coaxed. "This is your sister. I know what it is."

"I said I don't want to talk about it."

This was typical of Constantine. A bit of annoyance mixed with a dose of anger and topped with a wallop of avoidance and stubbornness.

I sensed immediately that he had been gifted with the same affliction. So rather than asking him questions, I decided to explain what had happened to me, including the limp, the visits to the neurologist, the muscular dystrophy, the tests to determine the cause, and then Charcot-Marie-Tooth. My brother uttered not a word while I talked. I suspected he was in shock and could not believe what he was hearing.

When I finished my story, he was willing to speak. Yes, he also had CMT and had been diagnosed in Florida. When Michel heard Costy's medical results, he shouted: "You're not a Malti. Get out of here."

That was the ultimate rejection of family history. I suppose I was fortunate not to have my uncle deny me my family name and throw me out of the house. But I was cursed like Constantine. The distinguished French neurologist, Jean-Martin Charcot, his student Pierre Marie, and their British colleague, Tooth, had become our lifelong companions.

***

Haiku for the Men in My Life

An Arab Christian,
I, a woman, broke all rules
Four men in my life:

One is a husband
The other three, foreigners,
Uninvited guests.

I have learned their names
Attached to the dystrophy
Feeding on my flesh.

Jean-Martin Charcot,
The most famous of the bunch.
His student Marie,

His British colleague
Tooth, the third to join the team:
Charcot-Marie-Tooth.

CMT for short,
Entering my life at birth,
Three men in a gene.

What a lovely gene
Remaining hidden for years
Until it appears.

Wrapped like a rare gift
Offered for my PhD.
Why that time to meet?

Inherited gene
Only allowed to exist
Through family ties.

One living brother
Absent from my life for years
Is my only hope.

Not part of *Star Wars*
No Obi-Wan Kenobi
To call for rescue.

A painful phone call:
Yes, he carries CMT
Is this Genes Gone Wild?

A chance destiny,
Powerful adversary,
Choosing weak bodies.

Degeneration
CMT's vampire love bite
Sucking life from nerves.

Yes, *les jeux sont faits*
Bodies holding losing cards
Failure etched in genes.

Nerves are bit players
In a game that is not theirs,
One they cannot win.

Yet they do not care;
Their myelin sheaths destroyed,
Quitting on the job.

Now free to relax
A long-deserved vacation
From pesky muscles.

No one asks muscles
If they wish to go on strike,
To degenerate.

But logic dictates
Muscles need a break from work;
May they rest in peace.

***

Constantine, it turned out, was in Mississippi. What was my brother doing in Mississippi? He told me: he was working for AT&T, but he had moved there to be with Mama.

"Mama?" I said in complete shock, not knowing what the hell he was talking about.

"Mama Odette, Fedwa," he replied with an impatient voice.

"What did you say?"

"Mama Odette, Fedwa; can't you hear me?"

"Of course, I can hear you," I said.

"Then stop asking me stupid questions." If I had not known better, I would have slammed the phone on the receiver. Instead, I passed it to Allen, who was shaking his head "no." But he finally took it and began to talk to Constantine.

Allen was much more patient on the telephone, most likely because he could see I was beginning to lose whatever sanity I might have left. And, of course, there was the fact he could only hear half the conversation. He began by asking Costy about Mississippi, to calm him down. He had not heard the name "Odette," so he began that conversation anew. Sure enough, our birth mother, Odette, was married to someone from Mississippi and had moved there with her husband. Costy had recently left Florida to be with our mother.

***

I was sitting on the bed. Allen sat next to me, putting his arms around me as I wrapped mine around his back. How long did we remain on that bed, our bodies intertwined? I do not know. What I do know is that I was completely overwhelmed by the news from Constantine and that neither Allen nor I had any appetite for dinner. Charcot-Marie-Tooth disease could prove a cruel master, harder on Constantine than on myself, but it brought me and my family back together.

We eventually went to sleep, and I awoke the next morning with the realization that I had to teach. My teaching career had slipped into a crevice in my brain and remained buried as I sleep-walked through that part of my life. I returned to the hospital to meet with the physician who had performed the EMG and gave him the news about my brother. Now both of us had a hereditary condition, and the physician was extremely diplomatic in advising Allen and me not to have children because I could pass that lovely gene to another generation. I had already made that same decision. As I write about these events, I have to remind myself that at the time I was also completing my PhD, and I was thirty-one years old.

***

Over that summer, we made the move to Charlottesville, Virginia. The university had housing for assistant professors on campus, and we lived in an apartment surrounded by assistant professors in other departments. After we arrived, Allen was able to garner a position as editorial assistant at the *Virginia Quarterly Review*.

I loved the University of Virginia. As at San Diego, I was the entire Arabic program and was responsible for teaching all levels. Nevertheless, I loved teaching smart students who were anxious to learn. I was invited to speak at the Jefferson Literary and Debating Society (one of their members was in one of my classes). Once you had delivered a talk at the Society, you were automatically invited to all their functions, including social events. I confess that it was at these functions that I really learned to drink. I cannot count the number of times I drove less than stone-cold sober from those parties to our apartment on campus. Fortunately, we always arrived safely.

CHAPTER 23

Mississippi

While in Charlottesville, we bought a Volkswagen Rabbit, our first new car. It was also in Virginia that I began to reconnect with my biological mother, Odette. Costy gave me Odette's phone number and encouraged me to call her. Odette? I was still having trouble believing that she and I were on the same continent. What would I say to her? Our last encounter with the coconut macaroons played like a film before my eyes. I realized that I would have to call Odette. Costy had referred to her as "Mom." I knew that was impossible for me. I also recognized that whatever I called her on the first phone call would be my permanent way of addressing her. I finally managed to dial the number. Her husband, Joe, answered the phone.

"May I speak to Odette, please?"

"Just a minute. Awedayte. It's for yew," he called out.

The Mississippi accent took me aback. Then I heard a female voice.

"Allo?"

The last time I had heard this voice, I was a thirteen-year-old girl in boarding school. We spoke French at the time, and I found it interesting that that language still influenced her when she picked up the phone to say hello in the American South.

"Odette," I said with great hesitation in my voice. "It's Fedwa." I had pronounced the word Odette in a very low voice, because I was uncomfortable saying her name. Had she heard that hesitation? She said nothing about it. Instead, she answered in English, but with a heavy accent. Some of her words were pronounced as though they were French. I do not remember the details of what we said. I confess that I felt like I was speaking to a stranger, which, of course, she was to me.

Opening a relationship with my long-absent mother was unsettling. She would call every few weeks. In one call, she was screaming that Joe was going to kill her.

"With what?" I asked. (I had seen enough of human nature not to ask why).

"With one of his guns, Hon." (She pronounced Hon as Hawn.)

"He has guns in the house?" I said.

"Yes, Hon."

I was shocked. I had grown up in Lebanon with a father who had guns, and I never thought much of it. It was normal in the village. But this felt somehow different. I was not a fan of guns, and having them around a house made me nervous. I tried to calm Odette. I eventually learned that such dramas were part of their marriage rituals.

Odette wanted us to pay them a visit. Costy dropped in frequently, but she had not seen me in decades. After many negotiations all around, we decided to drive to Mississippi and spend Christmas with Constantine, Odette, Joe, and their extended family.

Mississippi was far from Virginia, but we had our trusty Rabbit that could scale trees, as the salesman said when we purchased the car in Charlottesville. I was the driver, and Joe and Odette felt that it would be best for me to drive to a prearranged point where we would meet, and then continue on to their home.

It was dusk as we arrived at the meeting point, an empty parking lot next to an enormous building. We were clearly on the side of the building, since no doors or windows were visible. The area was ominously empty, except for a large American car with two people in it. We stopped and got out of our Rabbit as the two individuals in the American vehicle emerged and walked toward us. It felt like we were setting up an illicit exchange in a TV crime drama.

It was our family reunion. We all began to hug one another: Odette, Costy, Allen, and me. A group Odette would eventually call "*les quatres mousquetaires*" (the four Musketeers).

***

My mother drove, and I followed her. I had no sense of where we were. We drove down a highway a short distance, made right turns and left turns, then more right turns followed by left turns. My mother was driving slowly to make sure I could follow her in the dark. Finally, she pulled into a driveway and stopped the car. I pulled the Rabbit behind her, and we all stood outside our cars for a few moments while my mother pulled out house keys to open the door.

Odette kept looking at me, with tears in her eyes:

"You're beautiful, Hon. You're beautiful."

My mother was a tall, thin woman wearing black with her hair in a bun on the back of her head. I did not recognize her. She was a stranger to me. I felt obscurely that I should have experienced some stronger, more emotional connection, but all I felt at this first meeting was distance from this person whom I knew to be my mother. Costy looked very happy, and his dystrophy had barely begun to devour his muscles. He had grown even more handsome over the years, with sparkling dark eyes and an infectious smile. We stayed with Odette and Joe in a mobile home propped up on cement blocks. Neither Allen nor I had ever spent time in one before. The floors shook when you took a step. The walls of the shower were paper-thin, and you could make an indentation in them by pressing your finger on the side of a wall. Once you did, you were sure to get the weird sensation that you and the wall would be ejected from the structure.

We met the entire Rester family, including brothers, in-laws, children, stepchildren, and grandchildren. For a brief moment, I felt like I was in a scene from the movie *Deliverance*. We were the city folks lost in an unfamiliar environment, a place where older people have no teeth and where guns are part of daily life. Everyone wanted to meet Odette's daughter, especially since they already knew Costy. So we made the rounds. Most of the extended family lived in trailer homes minutes from each other. Joe made honey and showed us his beehives with great pride. The sociological disconnect with the elegant Beirut woman who had visited me in boarding school could not have been more complete. It contributed to my sense of separation from Odette and her family. This was a person I did not know and whom I would have to get to know, in effect, from scratch.

Guns? My initial reaction had to be revised. These people in the countryside lived with guns. Joe had an enormous collection, little ones and big ones—rifles. He had even taught Odette to shoot. Odette and Joe were wonderful hosts. Odette cooked practically all day, and we ate a variety of foods: Lebanese, mainstream American, and southern American.

One night, Joe returned from "poaching." I had never heard of poaching, but Joe explained that it was hunting when it was not the hunting season. Game wardens monitored the area, so the killing had to be done quickly and in the dark. That even meant driving without car lights. When I looked at Joe, I saw a ruggedly handsome man, completely unlike my father. Of medium height, he had the well-muscled body of a man who had spent his life at manual labor, with wavy, dark hair and regular features.

Joe told us how he and his brother were driving their truck in the dark, and Joe had spotted a deer and shot him. Afraid of the game warden, they threw the deer in the back of the truck, covered it with a tarp, and sped away. It was then that the brothers realized the deer was still alive. Joe immediately jumped into the back of the truck and wrestled with the deer as his brother headed home. Finally, Joe managed to kill the animal by bludgeoning it with a heavy C-clamp that happened to be in the back of the truck. He arrived home, his clothing ripped, and bloodied all over, including his face. My mother went into medic mode, cleaning Joe's wounds, wiping the blood from his face, and giving him a fresh set of clothes.

Odette was in charge of cooking the deer. Allen was excited not only because he adores meat, but also because he had never had deer so freshly killed. I have no memory of having tasted the venison. Allen found it delicious, and Joe said that "poached" venison was more tender than the meat of animals killed during the legal season.

One of the Middle Eastern customs my mother maintained was an affection for Turkish coffee, an affection Allen and I shared. He always took his *arriha* with a whisper of sugar, and I, *sada*, no sugar at all. One day, the four *mousquetaires* (Allen, Costy, Odette, and me) were all sitting around the kitchen table, sipping Turkish coffee. My mother and brother both smoked at the time, as did I. The three of us lit up cigarettes, trying to break the ice so thick I felt I was in an igloo.

I turned to Odette.

"Why did you leave my father?" I asked.

She looked stunned. She clearly had not expected the question.

"Because he was fat," she replied.

"Because he was fat?" I said.

"Yes," she repeated. "I never liked fat men."

Well, that was one way to end the conversation. There was nothing I could say. Papa was not fat in the sense of being morbidly obese. Yes, he was overweight, on the hefty side. But he was not disgusting like some of the men one sees walking the streets of America, their arrival preceded by an enormous beer belly. I often saw my father naked, especially when he took an afternoon nap in the master bedroom on the third floor of the house. To me as a young girl, Papa was handsome, emanating power and kindness at the same time. Odette telling me that she left us, a four-year-old daughter and a two-year-old son, because of my father's supposed girth did not comfort me, but I was afraid to raise the issue.

Another question had been consuming me for years: when was I born? No one knew. I had chosen from a set of available dates when a judge forced me to do so upon my becoming a US citizen. I was never comfortable with that decision. I hesitated over the possible birthdays, as Michel barked: "Pick a date, you stupid girl." I now know that failure to accurately record a girl's date of birth (as opposed to a boy's) was routine in the Middle East in those days.

Odette was my sole recourse. Her answer was not terribly illuminating.

"I don't remember, Hon. It was cold. That's all I know."

It was cold? Not much help.

In some ways, I left Mississippi feeling as motherless as I did when I arrived. My relations with my brother were less conflicted, but we were also still in some ways strangers to each other. Even in our last years in Florida, we had been living increasingly different lives, and I had no idea of his life after I left for Cornell. Constantine was not one to talk about himself. I only learned more about his experiences gradually over the years, and as his encounter with CMT changed him.

That Christmas, however, I could see that Costy had adapted splendidly to Mississippi. He was working for AT&T and was delighted to be living near our mother. He was more relaxed than I had ever seen him. He laughed a lot and had a gorgeous smile. We did not talk much during that visit. For me, the most important thing was that he was not the same Constantine I had known when we were living with my uncle, and that, in itself, was enough to make me happy.

CHAPTER 24

Funeral

Our return to Charlottesville came quickly with the end of Christmas break. Having reconnected with Constantine and my mother, Allen and I both felt that this might be the right time to attempt a reconciliation with my uncle and his family. On the one hand, I did not feel I owed my uncle anything. His last action had been to try to deny me tuition at Cornell, and I had worked my way through school. On the other hand, I suppose that deep down inside, I wanted to show Michel that he had been wrong, that I was a success, that I was not a *sharmouta*, that I was married, and that I had earned a PhD and a tenure track position at a leading university. After all, this had also been his profession, university teaching. I have no memory of the negotiations, but we must have arranged our visit with the family. We decided we would drive to Miami at the end of the school year.

It was a long trip, and I was the sole driver. I recalled from my uncle's drive to Miami that a welcome area greeted you as you entered the Sunshine State, offering fresh orange juice. Allen and I stopped, and the cold beverage was as delectable as I remembered it.

On arrival in Miami, we drove directly to a hotel not far from my uncle's house. After checking in, we called the house and learned that Michel was in the hospital. He had had a stroke (either that day or the day before; I do not remember), had collapsed in the shower, and my aunt had not discovered him for several hours. He was in a persistent coma. We went straight to the hospital.

As we entered the large, almost-empty room, I saw George at my uncle's bedside. We sat in a corner, away from the bed, not uttering a word. I heard George ask a nurse if his father could hear him. The nurse, looking bored and tired, glanced at the medical chart next to the bed, then moved a penlight rapidly over Michel's face and eyes and declared that he was comatose and could not hear anything. Her words did not stop George from speaking directly into his father's ear. He began a long soliloquy about how sorry he was, about how he hoped he had not disappointed his father, about how wonderful a father he had been, and what an example he had set for his son. He spoke of his current wife and how certain he was that Michel would love her if he got to know her. George went on and on, as we sat there trying to be invisible. This was, after all, a private moment for Michel's only son. When George finished unloading his brain and his heart, he left the hospital room without acknowledging our presence. I understood that he was most likely in his own emotional world.

After George left, Allen and I proceeded to Michel's bedside. I looked at my uncle's face. I assumed this would be the last time I would see him. He looked to me like his normal self. I almost expected him to start screaming at me. In retrospect, I understand that this was just fear invading my brain. After all, had I not been present when the nurse made it clear that Michel was comatose? I do not remember uttering a word to my uncle, and most certainly Allen would not have. We left the hospital and drove to the house.

We entered the house to find the entire family present—all of Michel's children and their spouses, Olga, of course, and Olga's brother, Uncle Herb, and his wife. George was going through papers in the living room. He picked up a bill for a minimal sum (my memory says less than $5.00). Then he turned to me:

"You did not pay this bill," he said in a loud angry voice, repeating his words: "You did not pay this bill."

I was furious. Body and voice shaking, I managed to get the words out:

"Listen, George," I began, my voice rising. "I sent any money I earned to your father because he wanted to be in charge of paying my bills. If a bill was not paid, blame your father, don't blame me. Don't go accusing me of not paying my bills." I was so angry that, unlike my normal self, I looked directly at George as I responded. Apparently surprised by my reaction, he said nothing and merely dropped the paper in the envelope with the other receipts.

Years later, Constantine told me that when I sent bills to my uncle to pay (with my money), Michel would start carrying on. He accused me of buying woolen sweaters for my so-called boyfriends. I explained to Constantine that I had gone to Cornell without proper winter clothing. When snow filled the Ithaca streets, I froze. Like many other co-eds, I went to a men's clothing store in downtown Ithaca and bought woolen V-neck sweaters to keep warm (nowadays, these sweaters are marketed to women as "boyfriend sweaters").

Michel passed away some hours after the hospital terminated life support. In the house, the male in-laws (all husbands of Michel's daughters) began to go through Michel's personal effects, looking for items of value to appropriate. Lee, the preacher in the family and the eldest daughter's husband, decided that he should take Michel's car.

George and the other males were ruthless in their disposal of his papers, but I happened to be near his desk as folders were removed from drawers and thrown out, and I spotted one labeled "Albert Malti." I watched as a male arm grabbed it and threw it into an overly full garbage can that another male relative then dragged into the garage. I watched as other important folders followed the same trajectory. I waited for a quiet moment and went into the garage and surreptitiously retrieved the "Albert Malti" folder from the garbage.

Thus I acquired what I called the "adoption folder," which documented both my father's death (it contained the letter from Hana) and the circumstances surrounding my and Costy's emigration to America. I did not look at the contents of the folder until I had safely left the state of Florida and returned to Charlottesville.

Despite this intense activity of inventory and disposal, there was time to make plans for a funeral ceremony at the house. Chairs were brought in from somewhere. Guests would be served iced tea or something else nonalcoholic. One of the male in-laws volunteered to go out and buy ice.

"Oh, no, don't do that," George was quick to object. "We can get free ice from my motel."

"Yes," someone added, "Dad would have really appreciated that."

The ceremony would be fairly elaborate. Uncle Herb, Olga's brother, was a preacher, so he would deliver a short sermon. Lee, Helen's husband, was a Methodist minister, so he would deliver another short sermon. Anyone who wished to speak could do so. George was quick to volunteer, and so it went.

Someone had found an old Arabic book. Since of all the Malti brood, I was the only one who could read or speak a word of Arabic, I explained to them what this book was. It was a hand-written prayer book, a manuscript, and they decided that I should read from it at the funeral. I did so and took the liberty of appropriating the small volume. None of Michel's daughters elected to speak.

Like most eulogies, those for my uncle were not distinguished by their sense of critical balance. He was described as a brilliant scientist, a wonderful husband and father, dear old Dad. Afterward, Uncle Herb gathered us around in a small circle to express our feelings about the deceased. Uncle Herb worked in a facility for wayward youth, and I now understand that he was performing a therapeutic exercise. I said nothing. But when it was Constantine's turn, he described in graphic detail the beatings to which he had been subject. None of the Maltis said a word, nor did they evince any surprise. I was struck by Uncle Herb's response. He turned to Constantine when he was finished and said: "And yet you are able to come here and show your love." At the time, I almost choked. The words seemed so smarmy and hypocritical.

Years later, my judgment has changed. Of all the members of that family, Uncle Herb stands out for his wisdom and humanity. Not long after the funeral, Uncle Herb invited Constantine to stay with him, and he spent hours talking with my brother, helping him to work out his traumatic feelings. He left Constantine a substantial sum from his modest estate when he died.

The reading of Michel's will took place in the small study Michel had built into the screened-in porch. George, the lawyer in the family, sat proudly in his father's swivel chair behind the desk. All the members of the family sat around him. Well, not all. Constantine and I were excluded. The will, we were told, was just for members of Michel's family (though, legally, that included us, for we had been formally adopted). This was not about money. To no one's surprise, the entirety of my uncle's estate went to his widow.

I will never forget looking out the kitchen glass door and seeing the family sitting around the desk while George sat behind it, legal papers in hand. That image remains engraved in my brain. Is it because it finally convinced me of something I had always suspected—that neither my brother nor I had ever been nor ever would be a part of that family? I did not discuss this with Constantine. Perhaps this was because of my own unease, or perhaps because he, unlike me, had maintained (and still maintains) contact with Michel's family. His conclusion, I decided, was his own to draw and not mine to influence.

***

Allen and I returned to our hotel room, and I told him that I wanted to leave as soon as possible. He could always read me like a book, and to see that I was boiling with anger did not take sophisticated skills. He suggested we have dinner in the hotel, just the two of us. The dinner, however, was not as pleasant as I believe Allen hoped it would be. I began railing as soon as we sat down. He was extremely wise and never contradicted me. As I write about the Miami visit now, decades later, I realize that what I was performing at that dinner was a mental enema. I expunged the hypocrisy of the so-called family, the sense of being an outsider, George's personal attacks on me, the greed of the extended family, and the denial of what kind of a person Michel was. Allen never interrupted me as I ranted. He understood what a toxic environment I had inhabited.

As we were walking back to our hotel room from the parking lot, I put my arms around Allen and thanked him for his love and, more importantly, for his patience with my anger that had erupted like a volcano. He just smiled and kissed me, telling me I had nothing to worry about, since he himself had been completely disgusted by my so-called family. We both laughed at that as we reentered our hotel room.

The next morning, we got up early, made love, and showered. We had breakfast in the hotel, relaxed over some coffee, then returned to the room for a last bathroom break. We headed home to Charlottesville. My anger had abated, and I was relieved, because the last thing I wanted while driving to Charlottesville was a car accident.

***

There is so much about my uncle that I still do not understand. Perhaps I was too close to him to fully comprehend him. Certainly, he had his positive qualities. He was intelligent, hard-working, and disciplined. He has a Wikipedia article in his name, celebrating his contribution to electrical engineering. His is a classic American immigrant success story. Perhaps I should be grateful he brought me to America. I have prospered here, and I love this country as only an immigrant who appreciates all it has to offer can. I doubt I would have found the freedom— intellectual, personal, and otherwise—that I have enjoyed in America in any other country, not even France.

But from whence came the demons that inhabited Michel's brain and so often took over his body? How are monsters born? Nature? Nurture? Nothing I have gleaned from family history provides any clue. Conventional psychiatric wisdom suggests that he did not start abusing people in his sixties, but he did seem to have a special attraction (if that is the word) to my brother Constantine. Costy once told me the story (long afterward) of one of Michel's visits to Lebanon (on his way to or from India). I was in boarding school at the time. Michel gave Constantine some kind of order that my brother did not hasten to obey. Michel immediately hit the young child and had to be halted by my father, who admonished him: "You do not hit my son." Maybe Michel was just waiting all those years for his chance. I do remember the letter where he promised to provide "a strong hand" for his nephew.

Some of Michel's qualities were more colorful. He was a miser. I fully understand the need for a man supporting six children (plus two adopted ones) on a professor's salary to be economical (even a professor whose specialty, electrical engineering, permitted extensive consulting work). Some actions could seem humorous. For example, when driving, he always waited until the very last moment before activating his turn signal in order to lengthen the life of the bulb. Other economies did not feel so whimsical. Back in Michel's house in Ithaca, when I was on the toilet, he would enter without knocking to make sure I was not wasting toilet paper ("Two sheets! Only two sheets," he would holler).

His immediate family seemed to find these traits endearing. At the funeral, they told stories, half wondrous, half amused, of his extreme thriftiness. And they gave him a send-off worthy of a miser. He was cremated, and they instructed the hospital (or was it the crematorium?) to dispose of his remains. This way, they congratulated themselves; all the costs would be covered by the Social Security Death Benefit. At the time, I offered to take Michel's ashes back to Lebanon and spread them over the Mediterranean. No one was interested.

Families are odd, and family memories odder still. Years later, some of Michel's children convinced themselves that I had indeed spread his ashes on his native shores. They told Constantine, who relayed this story to me. I know that never happened. Michel went out with the garbage.

During my last year at Cornell, Aunt Najla sent me a letter, asking me for money. Even a few dollars would help, she begged, since Michel was not sending her enough money to live. This was despite the fact that Michel was the sole heir of my father's estate, which included, besides the house, a farm with orchards, cisterns, and olive groves, all of which Michel sold, pocketing the money. Though I later felt guilty about Aunt Najla's situation, I took no action at the time. Working my way through school, I was not exactly floating in cash.

***

Miserliness is not really about money. It is about control. Michel was a control freak. The same qualities that functioned as virtues on a personal level—concentration, discipline, organization—became something else when he tried to extend them to his immediate environment. In Florida, Olga never left the house, except to walk to church and come right back. In Ithaca, Michel drove her to and from the house of worship (he did not sit through the services). Michel did all the grocery shopping in both Ithaca and Florida, deciding what to buy, at what price, and therefore what we all would eat. Every day had its appointed dish—meat loaf, chicken, fried frozen cod fillets—and each week followed the others in a culinary monotony. The meals were uninspiring, not only in comparison with the extraordinary food I had been lucky enough to eat in Lebanon, but even relative to average American fare. Of course, how could Olga have been inspired when she had no creative control over her ingredients or her menus? On one or two occasions, at the cafeteria where I worked in Miami, we were given extra, unsold dinner rolls to take home. I gave the plastic bags, each of which held about a dozen rolls, to Olga. To my surprise, they never appeared on the dining table. I assume she herself ate these rolls (the only food whose quantity Michel did not control).

Fundamentally, Michel belonged to a type I have unfortunately encountered elsewhere: the self-hating Arab. Whether because of colonialism or the immigrant experience, such individuals are deeply ashamed of their heritage, both cultural and biological, of their mother tongues, and their entire bodies. That Michel married the daughter of Swedish immigrants is not extraordinary. It is the American story. More troubling, however, was his insistence, made abundantly clear to me, that the only standard of beauty that counted was the Nordic one. Neither Constantine nor I, of course, could ever measure up. The best we could ever hope for would be to snag a blue-eyed mate (by a hilarious irony, that is precisely what I did).

Michel avoided the Arabic language like the plague. I never saw him read anything in that language, which also never crossed his lips except for his two chosen insults, *manhous* and *sharmouta*. We ate no Arabic food and listened to no Arabic music. When my uncle sought a bit of exoticism, he turned not to his home region but to India. He had taught there and served as faculty sponsor for the Indian students association at Cornell after his return. One of his proudest possessions was a letter signed by Mahatma Gandhi. (My uncle's admiration for the apostle of nonviolence leaves me perplexed.) Proudly ensconced on his desk at home was a hand-carved nameplate in a foreign script—Hindi, not Arabic.

The things Michel took from the culture of his birth were not its creative achievements but its fears and angers. This Westernized, educated, Ivy-League professor made his middle-aged wife wear dark sunglasses whenever she left the house, lest she flirt with men through her eyes. He suspected one of his daughters was not his own (and told her so with typical diplomacy) because she had red hair, though this should not be a surprising outcome when you marry a woman of Swedish ancestry. Michel's daughter reacted to this impugning of her legitimacy by making herself the family historian.

Beyond jealousy, there was conflict. My uncle played a leading role among those Arab-Americans who sought to block US recognition of the new state of Israel in 1948. Yet, he never discussed Arab politics or the plight of the Palestinians with me or, as far as I could tell, with anyone else in the family. I only learned of his involvement when I discovered the newspaper clippings after his death (and before they were discarded by his heirs). But if Michel was indignant on the newspaper page, he was silent on all such matters in his own home.

In his quest to escape the stigma of his origins, to adopt what he thought of as a white American lifestyle, Michel tried to paint himself into *American Gothic*. The result was a Gothic horror. Arab culture, like others around the Mediterranean, promotes a great deal of physical touching between people. True, you do not touch members of the opposite sex to whom you are not related, but members of the same family embrace, hug, touch, and kiss each other all the time. For the entire time I was in Michel's household, I have no memory of anyone ever hugging me (save Connie, once) nor of anyone else in the family embracing anyone. Michel Malti must have been a very lonely man.

Perhaps the most important choices in our lives are influenced more than we realize by family. Sometimes, the influence may take the form of imitation, and at other times, opposition. When Michel died, I had recently completed my PhD, pride in which was one of my motivators for reopening contact with the family. But my doctorate was in Arabic, the language Michel had tried so hard to drum out of me. I could see the relationship but conceived of my choice of specialty essentially as a reconnection to my roots. Yet, the subject of my dissertation was misers, specifically medieval Arabic books about misers. This was a flourishing genre among the medieval Arabs, who especially prized generosity and stigmatized avarice.

I adopted the thesis topic (suggested by Professor Bonebakker), completely oblivious to the fact that it was a direct attack on my uncle. Had I been even dimly aware of this act of intellectual defiance, it would have poisoned the subject for me. Instead, I enjoyed the hilarious anecdotes immensely. One of the authors, the ninth-century Iraqi, al-Jahiz, is generally considered the finest prose writer in the history of the Arabic language. It was a psychotherapist, many years later, who pointed out to me that I could not have defined my professional life more clearly in opposition to my uncle. I had built a life for myself. I had buried my uncle—or so I thought.

PART III

Odette

CHAPTER 25

Texas

During my third year at the University of Virginia, I received a call from a colleague at the University of Texas in Austin. He asked if I would be willing to come out for a job interview. I had not applied for the position. It was in modern Arabic literature, and I was a medievalist. The search had been fruitless, my colleague explained, as all the candidates who had applied had been eliminated. This is not unusual in academic searches. Different members of the search committee take turns knocking off the candidates until none is left. Lateness can be an advantage. I flew to Austin, gave my lecture, and was offered the job. I had made it clear during the interview that I was more than willing to teach modern Arabic literature and even bend future research in that direction.

I decided to go to Texas. The main reason was the presence of a large, federally funded Center for Middle Eastern Studies. Such a center, I believed, would greatly improve my professional opportunities and increase my contacts in the Arab world (at the time I had none). Since it was already late in the academic year when the offer came through, I decided to move the following January.

Allen, meanwhile, had completed his PhD in 1979, received a job at the University of Southern Mississippi, and was living in Hattiesburg, which was not really a coincidence: Allen is firmly convinced that the reason he received the offer (over the dozens of others lined up at the academic meat market that was the job section of the American Historical Society meeting) was that he was able to tell these Southerners that, of course, he knew Hattiesburg. His mother-in-law lived down the road in Foxworth, Mississippi. Assuredly unbeknownst to her, Odette had helped my husband get his first job in a very tight market.

***

I had not told anyone about my handicap while I was in Texas, but I had been petrified because the departmental offices were on a side street, and to get to the main part of the campus, I would have to cross an enormous four-lane street that was heavy with traffic. My dystrophy was weighing on me. What if I fell? The campus in Charlottesville was geographically much cozier than the one in Austin.

When I was first diagnosed back in San Diego, the neurologist told me I might eventually have to wear leg braces. That was a prospect I pushed away as hard as I could. But in my last year at Virginia, I was becoming unstable to the point where I was concerned my unsteadiness would be taken for alcoholic tipsiness. With the daunting four lanes facing me in Austin, I felt I no longer had a choice.

Virginia had an excellent medical school with a famous neurology department. I will never forget getting into the elevator at the medical school; as I was preparing to close the door, one of my colleagues appeared with his wife and young child and entered the elevator. It is difficult for me to express the anxiety I felt as they greeted me with smiles. I smiled back and pressed the button for my floor, paying close attention to the button they pushed. Thankfully, it was another floor, below mine. I stayed in the elevator and got off when the door to my floor opened.

What I saw stunned me. All I could see in the enormous room were plastic body parts. I wanted to run back to the elevator and return to our apartment. A kindly male wearing a white medical jacket asked if he could help me. I was speechless, so he asked me to sit down and relax.

"I'm sure you weren't expecting this," he said.

"No, I wasn't," I answered.

"We get a lot of that," he added.

I was fitted for plastic AFOs (Ankle-Foot Orthotics) that extended from my toes to the tops of my calves. Such braces, of course, required special shoes. I would have to say goodbye to all my fashionable footwear.

***

One weekend when I was alone in our apartment in Charlottesville before leaving for Texas, I went to the closet and took out all my shoes, from the shoes I had bought in Paris to all the Capezio sandals I had purchased in Westwood and loved so much. There were colorful, shiny leather sandals with two thin straps across the foot, ranging from yellow to green, and there was a pair of blue thick-soled sandals with long blue laces that I could take up the length of my legs and tie just below the knees. There were so many beautiful shoes, including lined leather boots that reached to the knees for winter wear and ankle-high colorful sneakers from my Paris days. I laid all these shoes out on the living room floor and walked back and forth, looking at them. Each pair held memories, some of which I could retrieve, and others that were lost. I have no idea how long I stared at my fashionable footwear.

Since Allen was in Mississippi, I had the luxury of keeping my shoes in the living room as long as I wanted. I would return, pick up a pair of shoes, sit in a chair, place the shoes on the table in the living room, and relive the events in my life when I was wearing those shoes. Only then did I realize that I had been living under the illusion that I was an able-bodied person. I could not bring myself to part with all this footwear that I knew I could no longer use. I kept the shoes in my closets for years, only finally giving away the last of them quite recently, after my retirement.

Before we knew it, we were heading to Austin, Texas. Allen commuted from Mississippi every other weekend and on holidays. He tried to arrange to give exams before trips so he could grade them on the planes and buses. We both loved Austin with its Country Western music and freewheeling atmosphere. It was also the home of Whole Foods, where we shopped when it was a single store in downtown Austin and where we frequently met colleagues who were discussing university politics over rows of cauliflowers and cucumbers. On the UT campus, besides the Department of Oriental and African Languages, I was also involved with the Center for Middle Eastern Studies (where I became the associate director) and the Program in Comparative Literature, where I was first graduate advisor and then director. While the Center was more useful to me in my professional career, Comparative Literature was a greater source of intellectual nourishment.

One day, after I parked my Rabbit, equipped with a handicapped sticker, in a handicapped space, one of my colleagues stopped me. "Oh," he began with a leering wink in his eye, "I see you have a disabled sticker. What did you have to do for the university parking director to earn such a privilege?" Wink, wink again. I was furious. I wanted to scream at him, call him an asshole, and tell him he knew nothing about me or my handicap. But I realized that I had been keeping my disability in the closet. With plastic leg braces, I could manage to walk reasonably well.

***

As befitting a major Middle East program, Texas had a relatively large Arabic faculty. There were three of us. A male professor, senior to me, and a female lecturer, junior to me. Both specialists in Arabic pedagogy (I was in charge of literature), they worked over the summers in Middlebury College's well-known intensive Arabic program. One summer, I received an invitation to deliver a lecture at Middlebury in Arabic. My visit would also involve meetings with students. I accepted the invitation, lest my senior colleague take my refusal as an insult.

The lecture and my meetings with the students were wonderful. The rest of the experience, less so. They did not book me a hotel room but placed me in a dorm room. The shower was a distance away. However, that was not the only problem. When I went to the room at the end of my first day, I discovered that it was filthy. The bed had been slept in, and the sheets were scattered on the bed as though someone had just gotten up from it. All that was insignificant compared to what happened to me before I entered the dorm room. There was no light outside the door, which was almost a foot above the ground (with no steps). The ground in front of the door was filled with large, irregular stones. In the dark, I tripped on one of the stones and turned my right ankle, which immediately began to swell and was quite painful.

I called Allen and told him I wanted to leave Middlebury the next day for New York City, where I could stay with his mother. As soon as I ended my conversation with Allen, I called his mother. Fortunately, she was home, and though it was late, she was still awake. I explained to her what had happened, and she was shocked. She could not imagine that a guest lecturer would be treated in such a way. She told me to come down to New York as soon as I could. She also promised to get me a cane from her friend Elizabeth.

***

I took a taxi from LaGuardia to Ellen's apartment building. It was still light outside, since Allen had booked me an early afternoon flight. I pressed her apartment button, and she answered immediately. She came downstairs, cane in hand, offered it to me, and gave me a big hug. I started to cry because her generosity was beyond what I expected.

"Let's take the elevator to my apartment and have a drink."

"That sounds great," I said. We did just that, and her friend Elizabeth, to whom I owed the cane, joined us.

Ellen's apartment felt like a palace. Its enormous windows had a glorious view of Manhattan. After my sleepless night at Middlebury, I slept like a log. The sheets were clean. I was able to shower, though my ankle still hurt. Ellen wrapped it for me with an ace bandage she happened to have in her house. From this point forward, I walked with a cane, in addition to my leg braces.

CHAPTER 26

Nazareth

The Center for Middle East Studies swiftly opened doors for me. During my first full year at Texas, the Center hosted a group of visiting Egyptian dignitaries: the President of al-Azhar University and leading poets, writers, and intellectuals. I was delighted to be their guide and chauffeur. When I visited Egypt soon after, they more than returned the favor. Poets, writers, literary critics, visual artists, and political cartoonists invited me to participate in their cultural life. Proudly, I soon added writing and publishing in Arabic (from Egypt to Saudi Arabia and Iraq) to my accomplishments in that language.

In the Arab world, what I wrote was actually read. In an Arab country I visited, I would be met by someone eager to discuss my latest contribution to an Egyptian periodical. I soon figured out that one reason was pervasive political censorship. When politics cannot be expressed openly, it seeps into poetry and the other arts, which are all the more eagerly scanned for political implications.

***

I invited the Palestinian writer and head of the Israeli Communist Party, Emile Habiby, to come to Austin and deliver a lecture. Habiby was an amazing writer, and in my opinion one of the top novelists in the Arab world. When he arrived in Austin, he wanted to stay with us. I offered him a hotel room, but he refused, so he slept on our living room couch. When we awoke the next morning, he was sitting wide awake and reading Italo Calvino, having pulled one of his novels off a living room shelf. I was astonished. He loved Calvino, reading aloud to us the opening as an example of a great beginning to a literary work.

Emile Habiby stole my heart. He was an amazingly magnetic individual, and he reminded me a lot of my father. I considered it a blessing that he shared our modest apartment.

***

A few years later, I visited Emile in Israel (we took the bus across the Sinai from Egypt). He told me that I had relatives in Nazareth—that there was a Malti family established there. After some hesitation, I asked Emile to make the contact for me. The last time I saw Emile was many years later in Haifa in 1995, and I was shocked at how he looked. He was emaciated and explained to me that he had cancer. He wanted me to understand that he had the best medical services Israel could provide, but that the cancer could not be cured. I told him how much he meant to me, and he told me to go to Nazareth to see my relatives. He called them from his office to tell them we were on the way.

Allen and I headed for Nazareth, after having called my cousins there who gave us directions to meet them. The car driving us would stop on a certain street corner, and my cousin's husband would be there awaiting us. We did as we were told, and the next thing I knew, we were being led to a home, newly built by my cousin's husband, who was a carpenter named Joseph.

"No," I wanted to say. "This can't be. A carpenter named Joseph who lives in Nazareth?" But life has ways of twisting your mind around. We entered the house and met my cousin's family. We could not stop talking as the television was playing a video of Majda al-Rumi singing. I adore Majda al-Rumi and told them so. They informed me that she was a cousin and, hence, by marriage a cousin of mine as well. I was having trouble adjusting to what felt so much like being back in Lebanon. Icons and religious medals were everywhere, as well as a plaque on the wall that explained in French that this family was dedicated to the Sacred Heart of Jesus.

I was awakened from my reverie by a knock on the door. Joseph the carpenter went to open it, and it was my cousin's sister with her mother. Allen and I stood up, with me attached to my cane. I looked at the two women standing in the doorway. The older of the two also held a cane.

This older woman stared at me with sharp eyes and asked me in Arabic:

"Nerves or muscles?"

"Nerves," I replied in Arabic.

"Then you truly are a Malti," she said to me in Arabic, this time with an enormous smile. She started walking toward me with her cane, and I began walking toward her with mine, and we could not stop hugging and kissing each other.

My cousin's mother, whom I considered a grandmother of sorts, insisted on sitting next to me the entire evening with her arm around me. Everyone in the house, I believe, was as moved as I was. And to think that Michel had dared to tell Constantine he was not a Malti because he had muscular dystrophy! I think Michel knew better.

***

My cousin proceeded to serve dinner, an enormous spread she must have spent days preparing. There was *arak*, whiskey, and local brandy. There was baked *kibbee*, *kibbee nayee* (raw *kibbee*), rice with vermicelli, and *kusa mahshi* (stuffed green squash). There was *hummus*, *baba ghannouj*, *mjaddara* (lentils cooked with onion and rice), and there was pastry stuffed with spinach, and baked macaroni, not to speak of all the fruit and sweet pastry that would follow: a plethora of dishes I had not tasted since childhood. I felt, as I have so often in my life, that I was living in a tale from the *Arabian Nights*. How else could I explain these wondrous events, these miracles, these life-changing moments?

We awoke the next morning and headed for my other cousin's house. She was clearly wealthier than her sister. Not only was her house enormous, but her husband owned a car dealership in Nazareth (if memory serves me right). We were to have breakfast, provided by a servant. Once again, that amazing fresh bread whose dough is tossed in the air until it turns almost to silk, kissed by a round oven, and then folded to be served—a Lebanese and, obviously, also a Palestinian delicacy. Fresh plain yogurt was to be eaten with scrambled eggs (if one so wished), hard-boiled eggs, fresh fruit, black and green olives, and pastries—the whole meal was overwhelming. I told my cousin that I had eaten so much the night before that I could barely have a bite. But she insisted, so I had scrambled eggs with fresh yogurt and that bread I can never resist. Allen, who never lets a good meal go to waste, did full justice to the offerings.

Borders and labels in the Middle East can be misleading. There is no real difference between Christian Arabs in Israel (normally included among the Palestinians) and Christian Arabs in Lebanon. Alas, we had to leave Nazareth, something my relatives could not understand. Why was our visit so short? Could we not lengthen it? I explained that we both had to return to our jobs in America.

***

Back in the mid-1980s, Allen was still teaching in Mississippi, and we had a commuting marriage, one in which he did most of the commuting. Allen likes to say that, having lived together at Cornell before we were married, we were forced to live apart an equivalent time after our wedding vows. One year I had a grant from the National Endowment for the Humanities and chose to spend that year in Mississippi, so Allen and I could be together.

After five years, I came up for tenure at UT in 1986. What I did not realize was that, unlike other universities, tenure and promotion to full professor at UT were evaluated by a single committee under the guidance of the dean. Like all assistant professors, I was nervous about my tenure, but when I received that coveted prize, I began to relax a little.

One day, I received a call from the Dean's secretary. The Dean wished to see me. I made the appointment for a week or so away. I spent that time fretting. Why did the Dean want to see me? Had someone lodged a complaint? All sorts of negative scenarios ran through my brain. The day of the meeting arrived. I walked to the Dean's office, and his secretary greeted me and asked me to sit down. I sat and waited in silence. Finally, the phone rang on the secretary's desk, and she answered it, informing me that the Dean was ready for me. She got up, opened the door to his office, and escorted me inside. I had never met this dean before. He was seated in a large swivel chair behind his desk.

He did not welcome me. He did not greet me. He delved directly into his questions. Who was I, he wanted to know, and how was it that I had come in as number one on his tenure and promotion list? I sat there stunned. I had topped the tenure and promotion list? I could not quite digest the information.

The dean sat back in his chair and put his legs on the table. He kept staring at me, and I felt like an alien who had landed on the wrong planet. I realized I had to say something. So I told him that I was an assistant professor who had just been promoted to associate professor.

"Yes, yes, I know all that," he replied. "I want to know who you are and how you landed number one on my tenure and promotion list."

"I have no idea," I answered. "I am as surprised as you are to have been on the top of your list,"

"Tell me about yourself," he said.

I rehearsed my professional career, which I was certain he already knew from my dossier.

"Are you married?" he then asked.

I was flabbergasted. The dean wanted to know if I was married? I wanted to tell him that my marital status was none of his business and that I believed it was against the law to ask such questions. But, hey, I told myself, screw the legal formalities, he was the dean and I was still an assistant professor.

"Yes, I am," I replied.

"What does your husband do?"

"He is an assistant professor of history."

"Where?"

"At the University of Southern Mississippi."

Suddenly, the dean put his legs down and pushed his chair closer to the desk. Now he was facing me directly.

"In Hattiesburg?" he asked.

"Yes," I said, amazed that he knew the name of the city without my having told him.

"That's where I'm from," the dean announced, a smile on his face.

"You're kidding," I said without thinking.

"No. I'm from Hattiesburg."

Immediately, the conversation lightened.

"Wow. This is unbelievable," I responded.

"Why?" he asked.

I realized then how stupid that must have sounded.

"I'm sorry," I replied. "It never occurred to me that you were from there. I assumed you were from Texas."

"There's no reason to apologize," he immediately answered. "Hattiesburg is my hometown."

"Have you ever been to Hattiesburg?" he asked.

"Of course," I replied. "I spent a year while I had an NEH grant living there with my husband. And my mother lives in Mississippi, as well."

We were now in full nonacademic territory. Then I heard the dean's phone ring. He picked it up and said, "Give me a few more minutes." Clearly, it was time for his next appointment. But he was not finished with me.

"The next time your husband comes to Austin, I want to meet him. Make sure you make an appointment with my secretary."

"Thank you so much," I said. "It was an honor for me to have a chance to chat with the dean."

He waved me off, as if to say, "Don't be so silly."

We both stood up, and he escorted me to a side door in his office that I had not noticed was even there. This way, I assumed, guests could leave without encountering his next appointment.

***

If I did not have muscular dystrophy, I swear I would have flown out of that administration building like a kite in the sky. I hardly believed all this was happening. I had always felt that life was full of serendipity and that we needed to follow it wherever it might take us. Having landed on the top of the tenure and promotion list, with a dean from Hattiesburg, was in my mind a serendipitous event.

I made an appointment for the next time Allen was due in Austin. By yet another twist of fate, his department had just published an illustrated volume on the history of Hattiesburg. Allen brought a copy with him to Austin. When it was time for the appointment with the Dean, we both headed to his office, Allen with the pictorial history of Hattiesburg, autographed by the authors.

The dean was overwhelmed with emotion. He began to examine the book and wax eloquent about its photographic content. Of course, he remembered this, and he remembered that, and he thanked Allen for this unexpected gift.

Then it was down to business. The dean, I knew by now, would not waste his time with niceties. So he immediately began questioning Allen about his position at the University of Southern Mississippi: Yes, it was tenure track. Was he working on a book? Yes. With whom had he worked as a graduate student? Eugen Weber. The dean said: "Ah, yes, Eugen Weber is a great historian."

The dean then addressed our commuting relationship, something he did not consider beneficial for either of us. He realized that it was not only an expensive venture, since one or the other of us had to fly back and forth, but he also realized that it was a distraction for both of us, not only in our research but in our teaching as well.

Allen and I sat there silently. Neither of us knew where the dean would go next. Delving into people's personal lives was something I had always considered a taboo subject on the job, but this was clearly not the case here. The dean's solution was simple. He offered Allen a lectureship at the University of Texas. Just like that. No advertisement. No search. No consultation with departments. The dean asked us what we thought. I was speechless. Allen, however, managed to get out some words along the line of how this would be a dream come true, how pleased he was by the dean's proposal, and how generous the dean was to take this step on our behalf.

This dean, not one to mince words or waste time, cut Allen off by saying that the matter was settled and that Allen should expect to move to Austin. He would receive a letter appointing him as a lecturer. While this was not a tenure track position, we were ecstatic that our days of commuting would come to an end.

***

Commuting had been a great drain on our finances. Allen calculated that between airfares, a second apartment, and an hour-long daily phone call (charged by the minute back then), his Mississippi job garnered us less than three thousand dollars a year. Now that we were together in Austin, we could buy a house, and not just any house; we wanted one that was architecturally interesting.

But buying real estate is not a democratic venture. Real estate agents act as social filters, making certain that special neighborhoods remain special. That translates into keeping the riff-raff out of exclusive areas. The first agent we worked with clearly saw us as riff-raff. I had already noticed that in Texas, as earlier in California, I was often taken for a Chicana. The neighborhood we wanted, Westlake Hills, was not for us, said the real estate agent. It was filled with "executive homes." We had visited the homes of friends who lived in that neighborhood, and our minds were made up.

So we hired another real estate agent. This one was more forthcoming. One day, she took us to see a house in the hills. It was a three-story house that had been designed by an architect and featured in a book, *Austin and Its Architecture*. The book remains with us, and I often open it to stare at the house that became our first home. We fell in love with that house at first sight. Rather than a traditional structure, this house was built vertically into the hillside, almost like terracing. Each floor had a view of the hillsides of Austin, and each floor had multiple windows that provided different views of those same hills. It had cantilevered unscreened decks that made you feel like you were floating in the air with the ground beneath you. The influence of Frank Lloyd Wright's Falling Water was clear.

Needless to say, we purchased the house. It was a perfect escape. I could take my computer and write on the deck off the living room. When I wanted to be closer to the trees, I could walk out on the open deck adjacent to my study on the bottom floor of the house. Since, by then, I could barely climb stairs, we installed a chair lift between the bottom and middle floors. The top floor was Allen's study and library. It was while we were in Texas that I was promoted to full professor. I was in my mid-forties. Now I could say that life was good.

Some would say I had it all—a good job, husband, and beautiful house. And I did. But one thing bothered me, though it should not have. Allen's academic status (and consequently his salary) was lower than mine, a situation that continued throughout our careers. I always felt that this was unfair, since in my mind, Allen was by far the more brilliant person (I thought of myself as simply hardworking). Part of it was undoubtedly our fields (the supply of qualified Arabists was limited, while French historians were legion), part also our differing work styles. Once I started writing a book, I was eager to get it done. My works came out quickly. Allen was comfortable with long-term projects that took a decade to complete. He never minded making less money than I did. Every time I brought it up, he would say, "It is not who earns the money, but who spends it." And, of course, we always shared everything. In some ways, maybe he was more of a feminist than I was.

***

The Austin, Texas we knew is still one of my favorite cities, replete with beauty and good friends. Our friends, while we lived in Austin, were not Middle East specialists. They were poets, novelists, painters, and other artists. Our world expanded tremendously, as we would sit over dinner discussing not only literature and art, but also the best places in the world to get different types of mangoes. At times, we would escape at sunset to the bars on the riverfront and meet with friends over margaritas. Dusk was the time when bats would make an appearance over the river—a sight to behold.

But, alas, good things in life never last. The academic climate in the university was changing, particularly in Comparative Literature, where I had become director. Comp Lit was divided by the same battle that was churning in literature departments across the country—our 1980s version of the ancients versus the moderns. One group stood for literature with a capital "L" and wished to concentrate on the great works of the canon. The other side saw literature as also political and wanted to extend scrutiny to works from traditionally marginalized groups like women, minorities, and Third-World writers. Personally, I have always felt that both sides were right and that both sides, again, erred by casting their opponents as enemies of culture. I remember one meeting I chaired at which I looked around the room and noticed one group of professors sitting on one side of the room and the others sitting opposite them. Neither group looked at the other. I was saddened by this division because I had friends in both groups. I did manage to keep the program from blowing up, but the split continued during the rest of my time at Texas.

Chapter 27

Indiana

By the early 1990s, I was in my late forties. This was the point in my career when I began to get unsolicited inquiries about jobs. Michigan, USC, and Indiana were among the universities courting me. The USC position was for a Saudi-funded chair. I flew out for the interview in Los Angeles. By the time I left, I knew this post was not for me.

On the plane home from Los Angeles after the USC interview, I pulled a pad out of my purse. Because I flew so much to attend meetings both at the Social Science Research Council and the American Council of Learned Societies, I had gotten into the habit of always packing little notebooks and colored pens and pencils. I would draw in the limousine that took me from our home in Austin to the airport. I would also doodle while on planes.

This time, however, I found myself not doodling but writing little snippets. My brain was pushing me to write a novel about academia. I did not know how this would come out. When I returned home, I began seriously to write a novel. I titled it *Hisland* (inspired by Gilman's *Herland*). At one of our get-togethers with our writer friends, a poet was shocked when he heard what I was writing. "But you have not been trained as a novelist," he said. What could I reply? That using criteria like this, we would have to dismiss all the great novelists of the world who did not receive degrees from creative writing programs? I laughed it off.

Around the same time, I got a call from an old friend who was teaching at the University of Michigan. I had known him while I was a graduate student at UCLA and he was a beginning assistant professor. "What would it take to bring me to Michigan?" he wanted to know. That was an easy one. "A good position for Allen," I said. I flew to Ann Arbor, did the interview, and got the offer. Allen, however, got nowhere—not even an interview—so I had to decline.

I received an offer from USC. At the same time, I was approached by Indiana University with a position as Chair of the Department of Near Eastern Languages. Allen would also be offered a position at Indiana. We traveled to Bloomington for the normal interview rituals and, in my case, a meeting with the dean who would be my boss if I accepted the position of department chair. As an administrator, my salary would be substantially increased.

Spousal hires are always tricky. Unless you and your partner are in the same field, the spouse's department, in general, sees no reason to do a favor for some other department. Departments are a little bit like families (and sometimes dysfunctional, too), and they want to choose their own new members. But the Chair of the History Department wanted my hiring to work, and she cobbled together a position for Allen, a position that could eventually lead to tenure and at least guaranteed him ten years of employment. His position at Texas, by contrast, was a one-year contract—infinitely renewable, but also perfectly cancellable.

***

This was one of the most difficult decisions I made in my career. Did we really want to move again? But the dean at Indiana was charming, and the offer was way beyond what we were earning at the University of Texas. Additionally, for Allen, it offered the prospect of moving up in the academic hierarchy. We finally decided to accept. It broke my heart to leave that gorgeous house in Austin and our many good friends.

***

Our move to Indiana was coming up with the speed of a racecar. We flew to Indianapolis. A graduate student picked us up and drove us to Bloomington. It had been difficult to find accessible housing. Allen had gone up a few weeks earlier by himself to rent us a place. In my absence, he made a decision that did not really work for me.

The house on the outskirts of Bloomington was the property of a retired Indiana University professor and his wife. They had moved to Mexico, where the weather was not so inclement. We met the elderly couple on our arrival, and they seemed perfectly nice.

But that house was an altogether different story. It was, to put it mildly, one of the strangest houses I have ever lived in. It was surrounded by acres and acres of land on which only trees lived. The house itself was all glass, with no solid external walls anywhere. An entirely open wooden deck graced the abode; in reality, it was just a wooden floor protruding from the house. I will never forget the elderly wife turning to her husband and asking if he remembered her doing dance movements on that deck while naked. Oh yes, he remembered. The bathroom was protected by three solid interior walls, but the shower stall was graced by a full-length window (not glazed), offering a complete view to any curious squirrels, rabbits, or deer.

An all-glass house? It had a basement with an extra bedroom and bathroom, but my muscular dystrophy blocked access to that level, so I was confined to the top all-glass floor. Others might have reveled in the openness of this strange abode, but not me.

***

I came to realize something I had never quite realized before. I had been brought up in a village in Lebanon where privacy was key (this would also apply elsewhere in the Middle East). You could not look into people's shuttered houses. I had grown up always feeling safe in that environment. Sure, we could climb up on the roof at night, but the roofs did not permit views into the homes. Only now do I understand part of my affection for our spectacular house in Austin. The stilts on which the house rested permitted limited views into our living quarters because one of its sides rested against the Austin hillside.

I could not sleep in the Bloomington bedroom with its glass walls, so Allen flattened some of our packing boxes that had carried our goods from Austin and placed them around the bedroom's glass walls. He did the same for certain sections of the living room that I absolutely could not tolerate.

We decided to build a handicap-accessible house in Indiana and hired an architect to create a design on a five-acre lot. It was all on one level, and it had high ceilings everywhere (Allen's preference) and modestly sized windows (my preference). We even put in a separate stack room, filled with wooden shelves for my rapidly expanding scholarly library. The house included a small indoor pool in which I could exercise since my dystrophy seemed to think it was a Porsche and could speed without risking a ticket, making a serious workout on dry land almost impossible.

CHAPTER 28

Crash

My twenty years at Indiana University showed me a side of people to which I wish I had never been exposed. One of my most distressing experiences was seeing faculty colleagues trying to destroy my graduate students. Some were effectively run out of the university (one went back to Egypt; another landed at Harvard). I had to sit quietly while people who called themselves teachers deliberately reduced my students to tears. This sport, which I liken to child abuse, is one I never saw at any of the other universities with which I had been associated. Two of my best students, after receiving their doctorates, joined government agencies where their linguistic and area skills were sorely needed. Both are happier in their work than any professor I have ever listened to. One is moving rapidly up the ranks of his agency. The other told me, "I would do this job for free."

A few years after I began as Chair of Near Eastern Languages, the dean at Indiana, obviously pleased with my performance to that point, asked me to take on the additional role of Director of the Middle East Studies Program. Back in Texas, the administrative assistant at the Middle East Center and I had become quite close, and she had been quick to relate the adventures of previous directors to me. The pressures of the job were much more political, or even psychological, than academic. The first director had kept a bottle of scotch in his office and sipped it throughout the day. He was effectively a nonfunctional alcoholic. The second director, who had been a highly successful scholar, had a complete burnout and ceased coming to his office. The third director was an Iranian who must have learned politics in the old country. After he left the position, the administrative assistant went into his office to clean it for the next director and discovered that he had never opened any of his mail. His office was full of correspondence that he had never bothered to read.

The fourth director was the one under whom I served as associate director. This young Englishman began his directorship fit, athletic, and nonsmoking. Before he finished his three-year term, he suffered a massive, debilitating heart attack. I asked him at the time if he thought the summer salaries he received as director were worth the loss of his health. "Of course not," he answered. The lesson should have been clear, but I was confident in my abilities. After all, I had successfully navigated the culture wars at Texas Comp Lit. I was not going to burn out. I was wrong.

My Indiana critics had a tool unavailable to the Texas tormenters: the World-Wide Web. My Indiana enemies were skilled at using the Web as an echo chamber, making local complaints sound as if they were part of a global campaign. The charge that offended me the most, which even today drives me to distraction, is that I abused my handicap. It makes me want to scream. These people have no idea of the constant pain associated with muscular dystrophy, or maybe they just do not care.

The general strategy of my censors was to throw everything up against the wall and see what would stick. Unfortunately, in my head, it all stuck. Were it not for the experiences of the Texas Center directors, I would attribute my vulnerability to coming from a culture with an emphasis on honor, in which a woman's reputation is judged not by her actions but by what is said about her.

The worst thing about the Indiana attacks was that they reopened wounds I thought had been forever healed, and revived monsters I thought were dead and buried. My uncle's words came back, thrown in my face, as if it were yesterday. "Stupid girl." "*Sharmouta.*" "You will end your life in the gutter." My career as an Arabic scholar—the rejection of my uncle's wishes, the refutation of his charges—now lay in ruins, or so it felt to me. This *revenant*, this zombie Michel, was running through my brain, cackling in chorus with my Indiana ill-wishers. In my darkest moments, I could even hear that red devil who had laughed at me while perched on the wall in my Lebanese childhood. I dissociated, I slit my wrists, and my last ten years at Indiana (I retired at the end of 2012), were spent inside a huge black cloud. I consulted psychiatrists and therapists, lots of them (I even outlived three). I took pills—lots of them.

***

Pills

Purple pills,
Green pills,
Blue pills,

Clear pills,
Pink pills,
Round pills,
Oval pills,
Thin pills,
Thick pills,
Gel pills.
Every Sunday
I fill my weekly
Pill container, now
Attached to me, an
Extra appendage.

At times my mind rebels.
Please no, no,
No more pills.

At times I feel as though
I were an enormous
Multicolored capsule.
Just pull, just twist in half;
Medical powder scattering,
Disintegrating as I do.

I refuse to take meds;
They deserve the toilet.
I scatter them
Around the table
In anger.

Allen picks them up;
You must take your meds.
No, I can't, I scream.
You have to, honey.
No, I don't want to.
Please.
No.

I'll shove them
Down your throat.
No!
I clench my teeth;
He is stronger,
Pushing pills
One after one
Between my teeth.
Then pouring water
Across my closed lips.
The water spills;
My clothes are wet.

I get angry, I scream.
Tired of playing games
With my brain.

I do not recognize myself;
I no longer know who I am
If there was ever a me.
It lies buried in a pit
Under deep piles of pills.

My face strains for air,
But I am blocked from breathing.
Bottles of prescription pills
Lie atop my still body.
An uneven shroud, eerie
Orange light emanating
From the plastic containers,
Growing deeper day by day.

***

My first psychiatrist thought I was suffering from depression. I did cry a lot, but her diagnosis did not fit what I was reading about trauma, depression, and mood disorders. I consulted a prominent psychiatrist in New York, and he sent me an enormous packet (seventy pages) of psychological questionnaires. His conclusion:

I was suffering from Complex Post-Traumatic Stress Disorder (PTSD). The doctor explained that my earlier traumas with Michel, the loss of my mother, and the death of my father had left me with a vulnerability that the Indiana events exploited. These Indiana campaigns had gone on for over five years before I cracked.

Now I could add more initials for the inhabitants of my body and my psyche. The good-old familiar CMT had a companion: complex PTSD. I went on campus only to teach my classes. I lived in isolation, a prisoner in my own home, which I left as rarely as possible. I took all my meals in my bedroom, where Allen served them to me. For many years, I did not even use my exercise pool.

To this day, I have no real idea of how Allen coped. At the time, my mind was too full of its own turmoil to be able to reach into his. My only reaction concerning him was the stabbing fear, a fear that recurs sometimes even now, that he will one day get fed up with my physical and mental handicaps and leave me. Blissfully, he never has, and in my saner moments, I know he never will.

Everything to do with my career in Arabic studies was now poison to me. I could not even step into my stack room, with its beautifully bound leather volumes. I recently donated my classical Arabic collection to Catholic University in Washington, DC. But, in truth, I had forsaken those books a decade earlier.

My brain still needed some kind of outlet. A saving grace was that at least I could still work, but not as I had before: joyously, continually, workaholically. Now my brain, like my body, fought against its own dead weight.

CHAPTER 29

Exiles

When I accepted the position at Indiana back in 1992, I insisted that my appointment be partially in Women's Studies. Was it a premonition? In either case, I wanted to have an alternate home in case Near East became unlivable. So it was relatively easy, after the multiyear campaigns, to move one hundred percent to Women's Studies, which was in the process of being transformed into a department of Gender Studies. I never taught anything Middle Eastern again. I worked with the famous Kinsey Institute on Sex and Reproduction and wrote two books about the Clinton-Lewinsky Affair.

When I wrote the first of these, *The Starr Report Disrobed,* a gender and cultural critique of Kenneth Starr's famous report, I called a colleague in the Department of Anthropology, looking for a first reader. Her husband, the Dean of the Law School, picked up the phone, and when I explained the matter, he offered to read the manuscript himself. After all, this was a legal document I was discussing. The dean liked my book, and my involvement in the Clinton-Lewinsky imbroglio whetted my appetite to learn more about the law. A few weeks after our earlier conversation, I asked the dean if there were some courses or programs I could take at the Law School.

"Take courses? No, you should teach them," he answered, laughing.

I found myself offering seminars to third-year law students on "Disability and the Law" and "Sexuality and the Law." Teaching new groups of students was exhilarating, and I was fascinated when I read, word for word, congressional statutes and Supreme Court decisions. At once illuminating and disturbing was a term paper I received from a law student who was about to graduate. "What a tragedy it is," he began, "that many a young lawyer begins his career with a lie." The Indiana Bar Examination, he explained, like that of many other states, asked whether the applicant had ever consulted a mental health professional, including any kind of university counselor. To be admitted to the Indiana Bar, the candidate needed to answer in the negative. I asked my Bloomington psychiatrist, who herself had been in and out of mental hospitals, about this. Such questions on licensing forms were common, she explained, and her response was just to lie on the forms. I found this new knowledge disillusioning.

I had been elected an officer of the Board of Directors of the American Council of Learned Societies (ACLS). One year, we held our annual meeting at the Loews L'Enfant Plaza Hotel in Washington, DC, just off the mall. Sitting outside the meeting room, I was approached by an elegantly dressed woman who spoke perfect English with a clear Parisian accent. She was, she explained, an editor at Macmillan and was seeking an editor-in-chief for a multivolume Encyclopedia of Sex and Gender that the press wished to produce. The vice president of the ACLS had pointed to me across the room, saying, "She's the one you want."

The editor and I became fast friends through our French connection. The project took four years; I had to coordinate several editors and hundreds of contributors. Sex can be a provocative topic, and there were disputes about what kinds of material would be appropriate (fisting, for example, was especially controversial). I learned from the staff at Macmillan that previous encyclopedia projects had collapsed when entire editorial boards had resigned in a huff. I was especially gratified when I was able to bring the entire project to fruition: four visually beautiful and well-reviewed volumes. This was all the more important to me since it demonstrated that I could lead a team of strong-minded individuals without anything blowing up in my face. Also a matter of personal pride was our success in securing the collaboration of the famous sexpert Dr. Ruth Westheimer. We met: two Macmillan editors, Dr. Ruth, Allen, and myself in Dr. Ruth's Upper East Side apartment. We were getting nowhere. We wanted Dr. Ruth to write a preface. She had no interest in a preface and only wanted to write an article. After the women haggled for a while without success, Allen turned to Dr. Ruth and suggested she write both: "Why don't you think of the preface as an hors-d'oeuvre and the article as a main dish?" Dr. Ruth accepted happily. Allen is of the opinion that Dr. Ruth, who is both charismatic and highly sexual, wanted to be asked by a member of the opposite sex who was younger than herself.

***

Doing my university job with the gorilla of PTSD on my back meant that organizational and bureaucratic stupidities others might shrug off over a martini after work felt to me like a kick in the stomach. In the law school, I had to threaten to cancel a course days before the beginning of classes in order to obtain an accessible room. After a few years with the lawyers, I retreated to my ghetto of Gender Studies. But even ghettos have politics. One year, a new chair of the department informed me that I could no longer teach graduate students. My reaction was a two-week binge of compulsive eating that left me twenty-five pounds heavier.

Feeling fully alienated both from Middle East Studies and Indiana University, I found myself searching for an alternate community. I was and still am an avid, if not obsessive, reader of crime fiction. I perked up when I received an advertisement for a five-day seminar at the Virginia Institute for Forensic Science and Medicine in Richmond. I used funds from the research budget attached to my endowed chair to attend the seminar, along with policemen, prison physicians, and others who are seeking careers at Quantico. For me, the crime buff, it was great fun learning about blood splatter and ballistics. I experienced a small personal triumph one day when we all filed into our seminar room after lunch to find odd paraphernalia laid out on the table. What could all this be, my law-enforcement colleagues asked, perplexed. I laughed and told them they were gadgets for autoerotic asphyxiation, S&M, and the like. They looked at me in wonder, but sure enough, we received a detailed lecture on sex and crime scenes.

I loved the seminar, but when I returned to Indiana, I felt just as lost as I had before. The next flyer to grace my mailbox was brightly colored and advertised a "New Directions Program" from the Washington, DC Institute for Psychoanalysis. The program, designed for psychoanalysts but open to others, combined psychoanalytic theory and writing. The two-year program involved three weekends per year and an optional one-week summer writing retreat in Stowe, Vermont. I joined eagerly, even attending the summer retreat before my first fall weekend.

I found the community of practitioners and would-be practitioners oddly reassuring. These mental-health professionals were often so tormented themselves that they could make me feel almost normal. One colleague, a PhD psychotherapist from Dallas, shot himself on the grave of his father right after completing his painful manuscript about his sexual exploitation by that same parent. Naively, I asked the director of the program if he himself had been in psychoanalysis. He laughed and explained that his first analysis had lasted six years, but that after a few years, he went back for a second analysis that lasted eight. Some time had passed, and he was now in his third analysis.

***

Uncomfortable with anything related to the Middle East, my mind felt free to roam other parts of the globe. I took a strong interest in the Mexican painter Frida Kahlo. Frida Kahlo is as much an object of popular—even mass—culture as she is of scholarly attention. In Mexico, they sell T-shirts with her iconic face and the words: "Amor, Dolor, Arte" (Love, Pain, Art). I could relate. Like me, Frida Kahlo had to fight all her life with a recalcitrant body and enormous waves of pain. Allen and I hunted down her works and those of her artist husband, Diego Rivera, across Mexico and also in the United States (Detroit and San Francisco). Allen loves to travel, and he shares my passion for art. I published a study on Frida Kahlo as a chapter in a book on beauty edited by a gender studies colleague at Indiana, and Allen and I gave a joint paper on her at a trauma conference at George Washington University.

In the summer of 2007, Ellen (Allen's mother) called to tell us that *The New York Times* had reported a Frida Kahlo centenary retrospective in Mexico City. We thanked her, bought tickets, and flew there. Some years earlier, during our first visit to the Casa Azul, Frida's house transformed into a museum, in Coyoacan, I had managed to drag myself up the steps to her bedroom, wondering how Frida herself had been able to do it. In 2007, I could no longer even attempt the feat and sat in my wheelchair, looking at the folkloric ex-votos Frida had arranged on one wall and the political posters from the Spanish Civil War on another.

In many ways, Mexico replaced the Middle East for us as a non-European focus. The country has superficial similarities to Egypt: crowds, poverty, and pyramids. Two important differences stand out in my mind. Egyptians, like other Arabs, feel no real connection to their pre-Islamic heritage. That is just something for tourists. In Mexico, the connection with the pre-Hispanic culture is alive, as are some of the languages. The other quality that attracts me to Mexico is a refined aesthetic sense that one can find everywhere, from the surrealist sculptures on the Paseo de la Reforma to the colors in a peasant woman's shawl in Chiapas. I brought this aesthetic intensity into my last years of teaching at Indiana, integrating several of Frida Kahlo's works, like her visually compelling diaries, into my courses on gender and the body.

CHAPTER 30

Odette's Story

If Charcot-Marie-Tooth disease reconnected me with my family, the Indiana traumas strengthened my bond with my brother and my mother. It was in Indiana that I developed a true and deep relationship with my mother. I confess that this was not an easy task. I would call my mother every once in a while and always addressed her by her first name, Odette. I appeared on television a few times to comment on political issues in the Middle East, and I called her in advance to tell her which show I would be on. She always gathered her friends around her and would point at the television and say, "This is my daughter ... isn't she beautiful?" I am not sure whether *what* I said on the television meant anything to her.

During those years, I also got to know Constantine better, gradually learning what his adult life had been like. In his early twenties, he volunteered for the army, and it was during basic training that he learned he had muscular dystrophy. Shortly after, he left my uncle's house, living on his own in a set of apartments in different Florida cities. For five months in 1972, Costy was a member of the US Secret Service, serving as a field agent. To me, this sounded romantic. My brother found it stupefying. Since there was little to do in the absence of a presidential visit, he and his fellow agents hung out in the Everglades and drank beer most of the time.

Constantine found his career home, working for AT&T as an operator. Among the advantages of the job was that he could transfer to any location in America (this was under the Ma Bell monopoly). He spent two years in Jackson, Mississippi to be near our mother before transferring back to Florida.

Increasingly, Constantine's work life was defined by the evolution of his condition. Like me, he got worse, but with one huge difference. As I lost musculature in my feet, legs, and hands, I remained otherwise stable. When I fall (which I do often), I go down smoothly. Allen says it is like watching a tree fall in a forest. Constantine, on the contrary, developed a pronounced tremor early on.

His legs shook uncontrollably whenever he stood, and his arms wobbled when he tried to use them. This lack of stability forced him into a wheelchair when I was merely walking with two canes.

AT&T found Constantine a model employee. He had a series of girlfriends but never married. Without any close family, he was happy to work on holidays like Christmas and Thanksgiving, for which he received overtime pay. AT&T also paid for his on-the-job accommodation, including a motorized scooter. The company made him the poster child for their enlightened policies, featuring him in newsletters and promos. Other employees, however, were not so understanding. They resented his handicapped parking space and on several occasions even keyed his car.

By his middle fifties (the early 2000s, when I was in Indiana), Constantine could no longer manage. At work, his back was hurting more and more, and he could no longer drive, even though his car had been modified to accommodate a power wheelchair. He filed for disability, asking us to help him fill out the forms. Despite all we had heard about problems with the Social Security Administration, Constantine was approved immediately. AT&T, which was downsizing its workforce following the loss of its monopoly, offered my brother an attractive retirement package.

Constantine's lack of stability eventually meant he could not live by himself since he could not, for example, safely take a cup of coffee from the microwave. He moved into the collective residential system called "independent living." This is a euphemism. The truly independent live on their own. "Independent living" is for those who require assistance with everyday tasks, like preparing their own food. After his retirement, Costy and I spoke frequently on the phone. Then Constantine began to fall frequently, often when transferring from the wheelchair to the toilet or from the wheelchair to the bed. He would have to call 911 to get someone to help him off the floor and into his chair. I worried about him.

My concern was also fed by darker streams. I still felt the guilt of Aunt Najla's admonition to look after my younger brother. My fear, which recurs with every worsening of Constantine's situation, is that in his humiliating dependence, I see my own future. We made a deal to check in with one another daily by phone. The problem came when I was traveling (this was before the ubiquity of cell phones). I suggested Costy call Odette daily whenever I traveled.

***

In my psychological distress, I began to reach out to my mother. I would call her at least two or three times a week and ask her to pray for me. Her English was wobbly, and I could not explain to her what PTSD was. All she knew was that I needed her help and her prayers, and she was happy to provide both. My search for spiritual succor became linked to Odette's religiosity. As part of her almost-miraculous capacity for adaptation, she had replaced the Catholicism of her earlier life with the Evangelical Protestantism of her rural community.

Odette explained that she began to speak to the Lord while in church. It was there that she got the Holy Spirit. The Lord talked to her and told her to use her hands to heal people. She was at once confused and frightened. After the church service, she spoke to the preacher. He told her that this was a gift from God. She returned home to discover that one of the girls in the house (Joe's daughters from a previous marriage) had had her tongue stapled by her brother. Odette put her hand on the girl's mouth and prayed, and the staple came out. Odette told a friend about the event in the church and its interpretation by the preacher. Her friend assured Odette that the Lord had chosen her and made her special. Odette says she told the Lord she did not know how to pray, but the Lord always came to her aid. She healed Joe's son (the girl's brother) and stopped the bleeding of a baby.

My mother saw herself as a channel to the Lord. I once told her that my right knee hurt after a fall. She asked me to place my right hand on my knee. Then I heard her over the phone, praying softly to the Lord.

> Holy Spirit. In the naaaaaaaaaaame of Jeeeeesus. She is my only daughter, Lord. It is in Your power to heal her. I ask for Your forgiveness and for Your power. I place my daughter in Your care, Lord. You can help her to heal. Thank you, Lord. You are the Lord, and Jesus is Your son. Please do Your miracle. You are the Lord.

I was amazed to learn that my mother could heal the sick. One day, she also revealed that the Lord had also given her the gift of speaking in tongues.

"Really?" I said.

"Yes, Baby Doll," replied Odette.

"That is amazing. Can you do it for me?" I asked.

"No. No, Hon. I can only do this when the Lord gives me the gift. I cannot do it like this."

"Why not?" I was curious to know.

"Because that is the will of the Lord and His Holy Angel."

"Please, please, Odette," I pleaded. "I have never heard anyone speak in tongues before."

"But I can't just do it, Hon. The Lord chooses the time for this."

"I'll give you five minutes," I said.

"All right. I'll see what the Lord wants me to do. But I need silence."

"Okay," I answered.

No sound was coming out of either phone. I waited patiently. Soon my mother's voice could be heard. I sat there in stunned silence. Odette was speaking as if she were in another universe. There were a lot of sounds that were repeated once in a while: kha, zut, tukh, ra, and other linguistic combinations. After some time, Odette's voice stopped.

"Wow," I said. "What were you saying?"

Odette sounded confused. "I have no idea, Hon. All I do is channel the words that come to me. You see," she went on, "speaking in tongues is one gift, and understanding the words is another gift. The Lord didn't give me that gift." I must confess that I was rather astounded. The sounds were not total chaos but formed a continuous sequence of repetitions that stopped at times, only to begin again with another sequence.

With time, I learned to respect my mother and realize that her life, like mine and Constantine's, had never been easy. Our conversations became more and more frequent. I would send her money quite often, but she never asked me for any. She lived a simple life and had built strong connections in the community. She had a sixth sense for people. Everyone seemed to like and respect her.

Odette already knew that I was seeing a psychiatrist. One day, my psychiatrist said to me, "You know, there are two sides to every story." I didn't get it.

"What do you mean?" I asked.

"Well, you have your father's side of the story and that monster Michel's side. I think you should get Odette's version." My psychiatrist had taken to calling my Uncle Michel a monster.

I decided that I had to find out what had happened between Odette and my father. It still seemed so strange to me that Odette would leave her children because of a dislike for fat men. It took me some time to work up the courage to ask the question. Then Odette said something that made me wonder whether she and I lived in the same universe.

"You know, Hon," she began, "they put down the wrong year for my birth."

"What do you mean?"

"Well, you see, they added ten years to my age."

"What?"

I was already reeling from what Odette was claiming.

"Yes," she continued. "My papers, they say something wrong. They write that I am seventy-six years old when I am only sixty-six."

"I don't understand," I replied.

"You see, Hon, I am sixty-six years old."

"Really?"

"Yes."

I was taken aback by all this. "I'm not sure you can do anything about that now, Odette."

"I know, it's too late. I should have fixed it when I first came to America."

"Yes," I assured her. "That would have been better."

As soon as I hung up the phone, I wondered about Odette. Could she be going senile? I immediately called my brother and told him not to speak to Odette about her age.

"What do you mean?" Costy asked.

I explained to him that Odette was convinced she was sixty-six years old. I had already made the calculation. Her numbers were impossible. If she were sixty-six, with a daughter who was fifty-eight, she would have had to give birth to me when she was eight years old. I could not reason with Odette. Besides, I felt strongly that if she wished to live under the illusion that she was sixty-six, there was no harm in it.

Weeks passed. My curiosity about what happened between my father and my mother had not abated. I spoke to my psychiatrist, and she reiterated her position that I absolutely needed to hear Odette's side of the story. My psychiatrist could still read my hesitancy. Finally, I asked her if I could use her name when talking to Odette.

"Of course," she said.

***

I called Odette as soon as I returned home. "Listen, Odette," I began. "My psychiatrist told me that it was very important for me to find out exactly what happened between you and Albert." (I referred to my father by his name.)

"Really?" responded Odette.

"Yes," I replied.

"Why?" she inquired.

I had to explain to her that my physician felt that understanding this event in my life was crucial to my healing process. Odette agreed to answer my questions as well as she could. Her story this time was a lot more detailed than the simple answer I had heard on that Christmas visit to Mississippi decades ago. In the new account, there was no mention of Papa's fat. This time, Odette reported that my father kicked her out of their house in the village.

"There were three women against me, Hon," she confessed. "His mother, his aunt, and his sister. They ganged up on me and made my life miserable."

"And Albert?" I asked.

"He was terrible."

"What do you mean?"

"He was really strange."

"What do you mean?" I asked.

"I don't know how to say it, Hon. He was terrible."

"You can tell me in French or in Arabic."

"I don't remember the words."

I was trying to understand what she meant by "strange" and "terrible."

"Did he ever beat you?" I asked

"Never," said Odette.

I was relieved. I had always thought of Papa as a gentle man.

"But he kicked you out of the house?" I said.

"Yes, Hon. It was the three women that did this to me." (I remembered the battles.)

"What did you do?" I asked.

"Well, it wasn't easy. I told him I wouldn't leave without you and Costy."

"What happened?"

"He wouldn't listen to me, so I had to return to Beirut. Then I came back with my father, my brother, and a lawyer. The lawyer, he was good, Hon. But Albert had a lawyer, too. And he had all the church officials. I don't know how he did it, Hon, but I lost you and Costy."

I could tell that Odette had started crying.

"Will you forgive me, Hon?"

"What for?" I asked.

"For having left you and Costy."

"It wasn't your fault, Odette," I told her. "But I forgive you even though there is nothing to forgive you for."

"You sure?"

"Of course, I'm sure."

"But you know, Hon, I watched you and Costy."

"What do you mean?"

"My brother. He drove me to Deir el-Amar every weekend. I went to neighbors next door, and they let me watch you grow up."

"Really?"

I had been in tears for some time now.

"Yes, Hon."

I asked Odette if she remembered my First Communion and the see-through gloves she gave me along with a beautiful prayer book. No, she did not remember.

"I still have that book," I say. "It has been with me all these years."

"I'm sorry. I don't remember it."

"That's okay," I heard myself saying.

Actually, it's not really okay for me. I find it difficult to imagine that Odette could have forgotten my First Communion gifts, one of which has not abandoned me since that day so long ago in Deir el-Amar. I try to think rationally about this. How can I expect her to remember when I myself cannot even recall who passed me those gifts from my mother?

My mother comforted me and told me she was so sorry. I comforted her and told her not to worry. We both bemoaned all those lost decades. Trying to lighten the conversation, I asked her if she remembered the coconut macaroons. That seemed to say something to her, but again she was not sure.

I had been told by family members, like my uncle Michel, that my mother married and buried at least three men. I asked her point blank.

"How many men did you marry between Albert and Joe?"

"Only one."

"Only one?" I repeated.

"Yes," she answered. "Why?"

Her question took me by surprise. I hesitated for a moment. What was the point of secrets at this juncture of our lives?

"I heard that you married and buried at least three or four men."

"Who told you that?" Odette asked, anger in her voice.

"Who do you think?" I replied. "The Malti clan. Did it matter who specifically? Though I think it was Michel."

"What a bastard."

"I know," I added. "But tell me, Odette, was his name Boustani?"

"Yes. How did you know?"

"Believe it or not, I have no idea."

Oddly enough, I have no idea where I learned that name. But when I had to fill out a form that needed my mother's maiden name, I always wrote Boustani, which, as it turns out, was not her maiden name, but that of her second husband.

Chapter 31

Saying Goodbye

It was 2012. My mother was alone. Joe had died a few years earlier after being bedridden for months. He had a bad heart and bad lungs—multiple organ failure, as far as I can remember. Now my mother was declining. I could tell. She would go to the hospital one day, spend the night, and then return home. Her health was failing, and I could not bear the thought that she might disappear from my life again.

One day, she called to tell me she was in the hospital. I asked to speak to the nurse, who said that my mother was in very bad shape.

"What does that mean?" I asked.

"I don't know, Hon," the nurse replied, with typical Mississippi folksiness. But she added that my mother had been in and out over issues with her heart. I told the nurse that I knew that. I wanted to know what made this time different?

"She is very weak, Hon," the nurse replied. "The doctor wants to keep her in the hospital. She is asleep right now, but you can try to call later."

"Thank you," I said, and hung up the phone. Something inside me told me that this news was not good. I called my brother and asked him if he had heard anything about Mama. No, he had not.

"She's very weak, Fedwa," my brother added. "You know that already."

"I do; you're right, Costy. But I'm still worried."

"You just have to leave it in the hands of God."

"You're right."

***

I did not sleep that night. The next morning, I received a call from Mississippi. A nurse was on the phone in my mother's room. She needed to tell me, she said, that my mother was near death. I was in shock. The nurse explained to me that my mother's heart had stopped and that they kept restarting it, but that it kept stopping again moments later. She added that this situation was causing

197

my mother great physical pain. I was in tears. The nurse passed me on to the physician on duty, who repeated her words. They wanted me to approve stopping the care, in which case my mother would die immediately. I told them I needed to call my husband and to please give me a little time to make this decision.

Allen had left the house that morning, before any of these calls had come in. I called his department in the university, and they told me he was in class. I begged the secretary to please get him on the phone. Soon, Allen's voice came on the phone. I explained to him what was going on. He felt that he could not leave his class. I was crying at this point, and I told him that I really needed him home because I could not make this decision on my own. He finally relented and told me he would inform the students that there was a family emergency, cancel the class, and come right home.

While he was driving home, I called Costy. He agreed with the physicians that we should not cause Mama any additional pain but rather allow her to die in peace. As soon as Allen arrived home, he agreed with Costy. I did not want my mother to die. I felt there was so much I had not told her. I felt that I had not said enough times how much I loved her. But the decision was made.

I called the nurse, who wanted me to speak to another physician. This one was extremely rude, saying that they did not have enough beds in the hospital for the people who needed them. My mother's death would liberate another bed. I was furious, but I realized the inevitable was coming. The nurse was back on the phone and explained that my mother would feel no pain as she slipped away. I wanted to know if she could still hear.

"Yes, she can," explained the nurse.

"I would like to be on the phone with her as this takes place," I told the nurse. "I would like to speak to my mother one last time."

The nurse was extremely kind, and she brought a phone she held next to my mother's ear. I began to speak to Mama, telling her how much we loved her and how precious she had been and would remain to me and to Costy. I said how sorry I was that our lives had turned out the way they had, but that she would always be a part of me, and I would never forget her. The nurse took the phone and told me that my mother was gone. Allen sat next to me and tried to comfort me. He called Costy to give him the news.

Now we had to deal with final arrangements. Costy and I decided that we would have our mother cremated and keep the ashes ourselves. The head of the mortuary assured me in a soothing voice that they had already transported the body. When he learned that we had opted for cremation, he had no problem waiting until we chose what kinds of urns we wanted for my mother's ashes. Yes, they were perfectly willing to mail the urns to different states. Yes, they would do anything to help.

***

I called Costy, and we decided that we would both get on identical websites, moving from one to the other, in order to choose containers for Mama's ashes. I was stunned not only by the variety of urns, but also by the styles. I would tell my brother which ones I liked, and he would tell me which ones he liked. It felt as if we went back and forth endlessly. One could choose more or less ornate containers. One could opt for something with an angel or other holy figure. If your fancy was a biblical quote, you could choose that. Or, better still, if you wished to show off your own wealth, you could store a loved one's ashes in expensive marble vessels.

My brain was not functioning properly. I had assumed that I would choose one urn and Costy would choose another. Urns came in different sizes: small, medium, and large. Costy decided on one small urn he liked, whereas I had chosen another style. As we were speaking, I finally realized that my brother felt very strongly that we should have identical urns, except that he would opt for the small size, and I would get a larger one. I could no longer think straight. Fortunately, Allen stepped in. He talked to Costy and then to me. We finally chose urns that were acceptable to both of us.

***

Joe, Mama's deceased husband, had several brothers, but there was one whom Mama favored: Eddie. Eddie knew about Mama's passing, but I called him anyway to let him know. Eddie wanted Odette's house, but Constantine and I were Odette's sole heirs. Allen and I agreed to sell the house to Eddie for the sum he proposed and give all the money to Constantine. I decided that I wanted papers and other family objects Mama might have had. Allen agreed with Eddie that he would fly to Mississippi to look for family mementos.

Eddie picked Allen up at the Laurel-Hattiesburg Airport and took him to the Hampton Inn where he would spend his nights while in Mississippi. Allen called me on his arrival, and I learned that he and Eddie would go through Mama's house the next day to retrieve any materials I might want. In addition, Allen would pay a visit to Mama's attorney.

I spent the next day at home. The loss of my mother was weighing heavily on me. When my father had died, I felt I had lost a part of myself. When my mother then died, I lost yet another part of myself. I locked myself up in our bedroom and spent the time trying to watch insipid crime shows on television. Allen called me in the afternoon to make sure I was okay. (He had become reluctant to leave me on my own.)

***

As I write this, I feel overwhelmed by sadness. Mama's death cut an umbilical cord that connected me to my lost childhood. I cried plenty when Papa died suddenly, and now I had lost my mother. I so wished that my parents' marriage had not been annulled. I so wished that I could travel back in time and begin my relationship with my mother anew. I felt so guilty that I had not called her Mama from the first moment we were in touch in America.

Only by setting words on a page do I realize that I must have been very angry at my mother. (I was never angry at my father.) I never understood as a child or even as an adult how my mother could have disappeared like a genie from *The Arabian Nights*. It took me years to turn that anger into abiding love. Now I can only be angry at myself for my own cruelty and for the hurt I must have needlessly caused my mother.

After their visit to the attorney, Allen and Eddie headed to my mother's house. Allen called later in the afternoon.

"She has a lot of stuff," he told me.

"I want it all," I replied.

"Are you sure?" Allen asked.

"It's my mother's stuff we're talking about. Yes, I am sure. Promise me you will pack up everything."

"Okay, if that's what you want."

"That's what I want."

Allen began going through my mother's house with Eddie, but he called me again to tell me there were multiple copies of the Bible. Was I sure I wanted them all? Yes, I repeated. I want everything.

Put bluntly, my mother had been a hoarder, much as I had been for years. She and I had never talked about this shared behavior. When we had driven to visit her when I was teaching at the University of Virginia, her house looked perfectly normal. My mother seemed happy.

***

I am only beginning to understand my own hoarding as I write about my mother. My hoarding began in a serious way when I was undergoing attacks and death threats while teaching at Indiana. I would order clothing and objects from catalogues. I became familiar with catalogues when we lived in that all-glass house in Bloomington. There, multiple catalogues arrived on a daily basis for the owners of the house. I had been blissfully unaware that it was possible to get clothing, furniture, soaps—anything your heart desired, even jewelry—by mail. When the catalogues first arrived, we just threw them out. When I needed clothing early on in Bloomington, I would head to the mall, where one of my favorite stores was The Limited. It had exactly what I needed.

It was only later, as my complex PTSD was coming in, that I went into isolation mode. Then I became afraid of seeing my attackers if I ventured outside my comfort zone. Going to the mall was out of the question, so if I needed clothing, such as pants, I would go to a Lands' End catalogue. And then it was on to J. Crew and Eddie Bauer, and from there to Peterman and others. I would not simply order one pair of pants or one sweater. No, I had to have multiples of everything. I would say to Allen that this was all just in case. Just in case what, I never even asked myself. As boxes piled up on boxes and accumulated under the bed and in the corners, whole rooms became unenterable.

***

The fact that my mother was a hoarder did not shock me. I called Allen on Eddie's telephone to tell him again that I wanted him to bring back anything of significance from my mother's house, such as photo albums, Bibles, jewelry—whatever he and Eddie found. I simply craved the objects that Mama had. I lived with the illusion that if I could see and touch them, I would somehow understand my mother better.

Allen called again after dinner. He had taken Eddie out to a famous barbecue restaurant in Hattiesburg that he had remembered from his teaching days in Mississippi. The food was still excellent, Allen reported, a sweet Southern style, and the meat literally fell off the bone.

I asked him if he had finished going through the house. Yes, he replied, they had.

"But, oh my God, you wouldn't believe the stuff that your mother collected."

"What do you mean?" I asked.

"She had piles and piles of empty plastic takeout containers."

"Do you mean food containers?"

"Yes. You know, the type you get when you order food out and bring it home to eat."

"What else?" I asked.

"There were plastic bags tied up and filled with plastic implements, like forks, knives, and spoons."

"Oh, my God," I responded.

"Even Eddie was shocked," he added.

"Did you take pictures?" I asked.

"Of course not," he answered.

"Why not?" I asked again.

"Because the pictures would just show piles of stuff. And anyway, Eddie and I are in the midst of dinner, and I am heading back to the hotel and coming home tomorrow."

I could not hold back my tears. Allen has always been able to tell when I am crying, whether he is home or not. How he can tell, I have no idea. I said nothing.

"Are you okay?" he asked me.

"Yeah, I'm fine," I replied.

"No, you're not," he said. "I can tell you're crying."

"You can't tell anything," was my curt reply.

"Please tell me what it is, Honey. Please?"

"You're going to be angry with me," I replied in a shaking voice.

"No, I'm not."

"Okay. I have an enormous favor to ask you."

"What is it?"

"Can you go back to the house after dinner and take pictures of the place for me?" I asked.

"But it's all garbage."

"Not for me."

"I suppose, if you really want."

"Yes, I really want. Why don't you ask Eddie if he can take you back after dinner, so you can take some pictures for me? Just tell him I'm crazy."

"All right," he said. I could tell by his voice that he was not very happy with the idea. "I'll ask Eddie."

He was holding the phone in his hand, and I could hear him asking Eddie, and Eddie responding positively.

"Eddie says it's okay, if that's what you really want."

"Yes," I said, "it's what I really want."

CHAPTER 32

Quest Romance

Allen arrived the next day, laden with stuff. Eddie also called to say he was mailing additional materials. What landed in my life was a veritable treasure, the likes of which I had not anticipated. I was glad my mother had been a hoarder.

I carefully went through the goodies my mother had kept over the years. The first things I examined were the Bibles. She had a number of them, one of which must have been her favorite, because she had marked it extensively. There was also a daily devotional in which she had highlighted specific passages in pink.

Mama also had an enormous collection of costume jewelry, most of which she had never worn. How could I tell? The price tags were still hanging on the objects, as if they were trying to make the purchaser feel guilty for having ignored them. There were necklaces, bracelets, and earrings. She had purchased much of her costume jewelry from Avon.

There was, however, a medium-size plastic box with a plastic blue cover that drew my attention. It contained round, gold earrings like the type I had worn as a child in Lebanon. There was more gold jewelry, including other earrings, in that box that I could have sworn came from Lebanon. But, unfortunately, I am not a jeweler and could not ascertain the provenance or the quality of the objects.

When Allen had returned and developed the pictures he had taken of my mother's house, I was shocked, but not surprised. My own area of the house in Indiana resembled many of the pictures from Mississippi, but with a different arrangement. There was a sense in which some of my mother's hoarding (though not all of it) differed from mine. In one picture, I can see a single bed surrounded by folded clothing and other materials. My own hoarding was messier. I was not able to walk into my stack room that held my books and research materials. I had retreated from my study to a spare room in the bedroom area of the house. That is where I would work when the cleaning lady arrived. The chair in which I sat and typed was close to the door, and I never attempted to cross the floor of the room because, put simply, it was littered with objects ranging from full purses to shopping bags. To walk through the space, one needed steady feet and posture, like Allen had. I once tried to reach the other side of the room and fell in the process.

Falling was not an unusual activity for me, but it left its toll on my body. The muscular dystrophy developed in such a way that I could barely hold myself steady without grabbing a piece of furniture. The floor of my workroom was much too crowded to take a walker through it. The walker would not stand straight in a steady position, instead wobbling as one of its legs would encounter an unseen object on the floor.

***

I carefully investigated the papers my mother had placed in a large envelope. Here, I found documents concerning the annulment of her marriage to my father by the Ecclesiastical Greek Catholic Court in Saida. This judgment of the dissolution of the marriage was followed by an appeal made to the Patriarchate Appeals Court of the Greek Catholic Church in Damascus, which confirmed the original judgment of the marriage dissolution. The two parties, according to this decision, "have the right to contract another marriage from any person they want according to the ecclesiastical codes." The document was signed by the Judiciary Vicar with the official seal of the Greek Catholic Archbishopric of Saida, Lebanon in June 1954.

This much I had always understood: the marriage of my parents had been legally dissolved, annulled by the Church. But the document speaks of an appeal of the original judgment to a higher court. The appeal must have been made by my mother. She was contesting this Catholic version of divorce. Was she trying to save her marriage, or just her relationship with her children? At the very least, this was not a consensual arrangement. At the time of this annulment, I would have been eight years old and well ensconced in my Catholic Boarding School of Les Soeurs de St. Joseph in Deir el-Amar.

***

My mother went back to her maiden name of Odette Moussayef, as she is called in an official document. In 1959, probably after Costy and I left for America, she married a man from Deir-el-Amar, Sobhi Ephraim Boustani, whose death certificate from the Maronite Parish Church in Deir el-Amar, Sayyidat el-Telle, she preserved. According to that document, her second husband died on April 10, 1964.

***

My mother sent me a letter by registered mail, dated July 25, 1964, to our address in Miami. Not only did I not receive that letter, but I only read it in December 2013, while writing these pages. First of all, I was never informed by my uncle Michel of the arrival of this letter. Years later, Constantine told me that he had once, while still living with my uncle, made the mistake of going to get the mail from the mailbox. Michel beat him and told him he was never to go and get the mail again. Constantine concluded that Michel was intercepting all communications from Lebanon.

I must have acquired the letter after Michel's death, since I found it in that old handwritten Arabic prayer book I read from at Michel's funeral. Only recently, as I was going through these materials yet again, did I find the letter from my mother. Michel had opened the envelope with a letter opener and carefully folded the letter and the envelope so that they could fit neatly inside the prayer book.

Is it possible that I could have overlooked that letter all these years? Was I psychologically unable to deal with it? As I read it now, I see that she had addressed it to "my dear children," though my name alone was on the envelope. The letter is in a clear, direct, even elegant French. I feel I must quote it in its entirety:

Beirut, July 25, 1964

My dear children,

Years have passed and ... still no direct news of you! ...

It is only with great difficulty that I finally succeeded in getting your address.

I do not know what you could possibly have been told about me, but it is essential that one day you know the truth and your mother will occupy, once again in your heart, the place she deserves ...

A horrific fear haunts me: it is that little by little, forgetfulness will install itself in you and that the image of your mother becomes progressively a more and more distant memory ...

Try, my dear little ones, to imagine just a little my present existence ...

After five years of Hell, my second husband, an alcoholic old brute, died a few months ago, leaving me only with bad memories and ... debts ...

During these sweltering Beirut summer nights, during which I manage less and less to sleep, my thoughts turn constantly to you: How are my dear children, what is their life like, do they still think about me? Are they happy, at least? ...

I beg you, answer me quickly, send me some recent pictures of you ...

I have no one else but you to live for ... I hope to find a way to see you again ...

I live now in the expectation of hearing from you, and, meanwhile, through my thoughts, I kiss you desperately, maternally, with all my heart and all my soul.

Your mom who has never forgotten you

Four years after the date on this letter, in 1968, my mother's "hope to find a way to see" her two children again took form. I can imagine my mother in Beirut, asking herself what the best hope would be. Clearly, there could have been no better option than to marry an American who would take her to America. Mama was undertaking what in literature we call a quest romance, which she followed step by step until she reached her goal. Her grail was her two children.

But how to meet Americans? Her best hope would be Americans working in the Gulf, taking R & R in Beirut. And so it was that my mother registered herself on February 2, 1968 as a "bar maid" (that is the Arabic title). She had to get what the French call a "*livret de travail*," an employment notebook with her picture, her name, the name of her father, the name of her mother (Fadwa, after whom I was named), her date and place of birth, her occupation, and her nationality.

How fortunate that my mother was a hoarder. This unpretentious little cardboard notebook, its binding reinforced with scotch tape, was among the objects she left behind after her death. When it arrived, along with her other materials, I had to decipher it with Allen's help. As a French historian, he was familiar with this type of official work record.

I began going through it, as one goes through a precious manuscript. I noticed that my mother changed bars quite often. She started working at a bar called ZIGZAG beginning on February 2, 1968, when she had her picture taken while standing in front of the open door of the establishment. Unlike in some of her other pictures from that period, she looks happy.

This precious booklet tracks my mother's life as she hopped from bar to bar, working longer at one bar than at another. Each page contains an official government stamp as well as specifying the identical conditions of work, no matter what the bar: that she not socialize with the clients, that she not sit with them, that she not drink alcohol, and so on. The registry for the last bar in which she worked, Crazy Bar, has her registered to work for three months beginning on June 5, 1972 and ending on September 4, 1972.

My mother's marriage certificate to Joe Rester is dated September 6, 1972. I assume Mama met Joe at the Crazy Bar. At that time, he and one of his brothers were working on oil rigs in the Persian Gulf and took their vacations in Lebanon. And so it became possible for my mother to get a Lebanese passport valid for three years under her married name, Rester, on November 18, 1972.

Thus, by the end of 1972, Mama, after years of trying, arrived at the land of her children. Only a few months later (at the end of 1972 or in early 1973), she and Costy found each other. Her reunion with her daughter (me) came four years after that.

***

I found it ironic that my Lebanese mother and I would end up sharing something more than mere genetics. I had worked my way through college waiting tables. I served people alcohol, much as my mother had done. I suppose that I should take my uncle's having called me a *sharmouta* as a badge of honor, since he did the same with Mama Odette.

PART IV

Mimo

CHAPTER 33

Facebook

Reconnection with Constantine and my mother did not mean that I forgot my Lebanese family. Constantine often spoke of our half-sister Mimo, with whom he had spent more time than I had, since I was in boarding school during her first years. Over the decades, I made unsuccessful attempts to locate Mimo. I later found out that when a friend of Mimo's, who was visiting the United States, called my uncle's house, he hung up on her. Odette was even more estranged from Lebanon than I was and was reluctant even to talk about the old country. Adding to my discouragement was the Lebanese Civil War that broke out in 1975 and has continued with fits and starts to the present.

Once—I believe it was around 1990—I found myself attending an official dinner at the American Council of Learned Societies in an enormous dining room in Philadelphia. The woman serving our table—middle-aged, friendly, and talkative—went out of her way to be nice to me. She asked where I was from. She told me she knew a married Lebanese woman in the Philadelphia suburb where she lived who looked just like me. I asked her the name of the woman, and she told me it was Mary. Could this be, I wondered, an English rendering of Marie-Noëlle (Mimo's name)? I could have jumped out of my seat and hugged the server.

"Do you know the family?" she asked.

"No, I don't," I responded.

She asked for my card and promised to contact me in case the woman turned out to be my long-lost sister. As soon as I returned to my hotel room, I called Allen in Austin (we were both teaching at the University of Texas by this time). He was as excited as I was. But alas, that tantalizing dialogue in Philadelphia was a dead end.

As the Internet emerged in the waning years of the twentieth century, Costy and I both searched the Web for Mimo in vain. We were both disappointed and finally gave up on ever finding whoever remained of our relatives in Lebanon.

Then the Bennington Writing Seminars entered my life. As the holder of an endowed chair in the College of Arts and Sciences at Indiana University, I had been blessed with a generous research budget. I decided to put some of that money to good use by undertaking an MFA in creative writing. I applied to three different programs and was accepted in all three, but settled on Bennington, beginning in 2009. Their low residency program meant that I only needed to be absent for one week at the beginning of the semester and one week in the summer. I began giving words to my adventures in Middle Eastern studies, but after two months, I came to the realization that that was not where I should direct my writing.

Instead, I took off on a project I had begun when Allen and I were fellows at the Rockefeller Foundation Center in Bellagio, Italy, in 1992, about reviving my Lebanese childhood. Among the fellows who shared the villa was Henry Louis "Skip" Gates Jr. I was completing a book on the Egyptian feminist writer, Dr. Nawal el-Saadawi, and Allen was working on a book on the French newspaper *Le Canard Enchaîné*. Skip Gates was writing his memoirs, and he kept the FedEx office in Bellagio quite busy as his words raced from Italy to America and back.

Fellows were invited to give readings from their work to the other residents. I was placed alongside Skip for the evening and knew he would be reading from his memoirs. I decided to read a short piece about my Aunt Najla to accompany Skip's telling of his own childhood. He read first, and I followed. The outpouring of emotion that greeted Skip's reading extended to mine. I remember sitting in the library at the Villa Serbelloni as the resident fellows and their partners hugged me.

Writing those chapters about my childhood for the Bennington program stirred something. After I submitted my packet for the January 2010 residency, I turned again to the Web, and once more googled "Marie-Noelle Malti." To my astonishment, a Marie-Noelle Malti Zakhour was on Facebook. I sent a simple email to the address: "Are you by any chance," I asked, "the daughter of Dr. Albert Malti from the village of Deir el-Amar?" With no answer to my email and my upcoming departure for Bennington, I resorted to calling my brother. I heard his voice from Florida as I told him what I had discovered and passed him the email address. Costy responded as usual: he was tired, and he could not commit himself to anything. I went off to the wintry world of Bennington, Vermont.

Allen arrived to pick me up after one of the workshops, and the first words out of his mouth were that Costy had been in touch with our sister, Mimo. We headed as fast as he could push the wheelchair through the snow to my dorm room. I called Costy, and we were both overcome with emotion. Months before they sparked the Arab Spring, Google and Facebook had just reunited my family. Mimo had answered an email from Constantine, and they had already spoken at length. He gave me her phone number in Lebanon, and I promised to call him back as soon as I had spoken to her. Hands shaking, I asked Allen to dial the number in Beirut. He passed me the iPhone as the ringing in Lebanon began. I heard Mimo's voice, and she and I broke into tears. We had all been crying when Costy and I left Lebanon more than fifty years before, and hearing her voice after half a century, it was as if our tears had never ceased, as if I were magically transported to that moment when Costy and I parted from both our native land and our sister.

Hours on the phone in Bennington with family members could not begin to fill the emotional chasm created by years of separation. Mimo was as moved as I was. Allen and I decided to go to Lebanon as soon as we could—the country was experiencing a period of calm, and we planned the trip for the coming September, 2010. We invited Costy along, but his increasing disability (much worse than mine) would make such a journey especially arduous, and he elected not to join us.

Chapter 34

La Yadum Ightirabi
(My Exile Will Not Last)

A heavenly voice native to Lebanon,
Fairuz,
Serenades me on the plane to Beirut.

The night before in a Chicago hotel room,
Eyes wandering over Lake Michigan,
I dial my brother's number in Florida.
Inadvertently calling him Tino,
His long-ago name.

My sister, Mimo, Allen says,
Has already changed our lives.
Am I not calling Costy Tino?

Costy's voice reaches me through the telephone,
"Oh, my God. I can't believe this.
You sound just like Mimo."
"We all sound like each other," I reply.

Strange feelings I cannot identify,
Being here—or is it being there
Or maybe even nowhere
Floating over the Atlantic?
Hours later floating over the Mediterranean.

Fairuz enters my ears through Air France headphones,
La Yadum Ightirabi
(My Exile Will Not Last).
I close my eyes
Traveling back into an alien space
Lost between no time and no time,
Between nowhere and nowhere.

La Yadum Ightirabi—Fairuz leads me by the hand,
Somewhere I find myself falling
Only to be saved by her voice,
Bringing tears to my eyes
Clouding my vision.
As the plane begins its descent to Beirut,
City lights merge in my blurred view
With the Mediterranean.

Mimo promises to greet us at the airport,
Carrying a sign with our names.
    She says security restrictions limit access
    To her and her husband only,
    Lest I forget my native land
        Is a land of war.

I await the wheelchair to carry me
From the plane to the airport.
    An elderly gentleman arrives to wheel me;
    Dignity emanates from his appearance.
    He smiles at me,
Speaks to me in Arabic.
He asks about our visit
Hears about the family reunion
After more than fifty years.
His face lights up
He finds the story entrancing.
He welcomes me over and over again.

How I have missed the human warmth of Lebanese hospitality.
My heart opens to this gentleman
Dedicating himself to making me
Feel at home, feel welcome.
Does he remind me of my father
With his warm, round face?
His having to wheel me mortifies me
I tell myself it should be the reverse.
Should I not show my respect by
Offering him the wheelchair instead?

Why is everything moving at a snail's pace?
Cripples are wheeled off first,
But we must await a special door
Suspended in a no-man's land
    Between jet way and world,
    Nothing to do but watch passengers file by.

Do I hear the elderly gentleman, hands on my wheelchair,
Whisper the words "Open Sesame?"
I am surely hallucinating.
At last the locks are released,
The magical door opens.
I breathe a sigh of relief.
Entering an enormous empty room
Shuttered duty-free shops,
Young soldiers seriously armed,
Standing at attention,
Eyes boring through every traveler
Assessing body movements
No humor in their demeanor.
    I move effortlessly
    As if I belong in this country.

Allen, anxious, looking at the rolling belt
    Moving round and round,
    A dizzying display
    Of overweight suitcases,
    Taped boxes ready to burst
    On the endless curves
    Of that enormous, wide-bodied snake.
    A slithering jungle of luggage
    Mindlessly repeating its journey
    As though it had lost
    All sense of direction.

Glued to my wheelchair, I also gaze at the rolling belt;
I spot suitcases Allen has missed.
    Is this not to be expected?
    Is he not more exhausted than I am?
    Traveling with a crip is no holiday,
    The constant fear I'll fall
    (which I often do).
    I do not make a very good cripple
    Always pushing my body to the edge
    Too impatient to follow
    My therapist's instructions
    How to move without falling.

The wheelchair advances.
    An enormous group of people in the distance
    Do I see a sign?
    My eyes could be fooling me
    Fear of disappointing my long-lost family
    Has robbed me of sleep for two days.
    But, no, I am not delirious;
    There is a sign
    I point to it.

We approach the crowd gathered as one colorful body.
A woman in a light blue dress steps out
Offers a bouquet of flowers,
    Swimming with red roses,
A multicolor mylar "welcome" balloon.

She waves, I wave, time stops.
She hugs me, bent over my wheelchair.
I wrap my arms around her as if she were a life raft.
Tall, strong. Charcot has spared her.

I keep mumbling "Mimo"—she keeps mumbling "Fedwa."
Not the three-year old I left;
An elegant woman
Large dark eyes awash with tears
Long black hair sparkling with stray drops.

The wheelchair moves, holding our merged bodies.

I am suddenly aware the immense crowd gathered
Is there to welcome us.
Cameras flashing,
Videotapes rolling,
A historic encounter,
    Reunion immortalized.

My shame at being a cripple
Keeps knocking.
I attempt to keep it locked in its closet,
But, alas, there is no escape.
These videotapes in the Beirut airport
Permanent testimony to my strangeness.

Slowly, slowly, we approach the mass of people;
I now see individuals,
So many,
So many I cannot count.
Cheering, smiling,
Male and female voices,
All speaking at once, crying at once, calling our names at once.

So many embraces
Surround me in my wheelchair.
Have I ever felt so much affection?

I do not recognize anyone;
I barely recognize myself.
Where is Allen?
He is equally surrounded
By family too many to count
Hugging him, welcoming him.
Testifying to the existence
Of my Lebanese self
Buried for over fifty years.

A glance at Allen's face tells me he is worried.
I ask what is wrong.
"We didn't get visas."
We were told visas were mandatory;
Allen fears we may not be able
To leave the country.

Mimo's husband, Halim, has a sixth sense,
Becoming aware
That something is amiss.
He examines
The passports page by page,
Spotting the Lebanese entry stamps,
Carefully showing them to Allen.
"What about the visas?" Asks Allen
Halim laughs;
The entry stamp is the only requirement.

Leaving the airport, I feel again like a burden,
A rented wheelchair
Reluctantly greeting me,
My permanent companion
During my stay in Lebanon.
But first a game of switcheroo
    As both Halim and Allen help me
    Transfer my body
    From the airport wheelchair
    To the rented one.
        I keep repeating my mantra
        "I'm sorry, I'm sorry, I'm sorry."
        But this time in Lebanese dialect
        Having sat for so long on airplanes
        In airport lounges.
        My standing body is wobbling jello;
        I must keep from spilling all over the ground.

I enter Halim's van, wheelchair in the trunk,
Body in the front passenger seat.
Allen in the seat behind me, Mimo by his side.

The welcoming party disperses to different vehicles;
I cannot count the cars.
Whatever part of my brain still functions
Tells me we are beginning
A veritable procession
To Mansouria,
The area of Beirut
Where my family lives.

Halim leads the parade,
Cell phone attached to his ear,
Guiding and directing the line of cars.

I have been wandering, searching,

Lost in time and space,
Existence suspended
In an alien environment,
My senses starved.

Hungry beggar at a feast,
I cannot turn away
From the smells of my childhood
I never dreamt of encountering again.
Provocative advertisements
Speak to Beirut's openness.
Political posters remind me
My native land has many faiths.
Neon restaurant lights,
People of all ages in the streets.

My mind races, unable to block the questions plaguing me:
Is it possible to retrieve a lost self?
Is it possible to reverse time?
Is it possible to begin life anew?

In my head, Fairuz's voice still echoes:

La Yadum Ightirabi,
La Yadum Ightirabi,
La Yadum Ightirabi.

CHAPTER 35

Family

At last, we arrived. I stared at the door before we entered the building. Religious icons greeted me. Everyone from the airport had somehow managed to join us at Mimo's house. I was still carrying the mylar balloon. I felt like a freak, everyone around me able-bodied. I was transferred out of the wheelchair as I got into Halim's van and back into the wheelchair as we entered the elevator to get to the third floor of their home. We finally arrived in Mimo's living room. She and her husband live in an enormous section of a three-floor building.

At the late night supper, I had trouble sorting out all the relatives and in-laws. Not so with Mimo and Halim's three children. My brain imprinted them quickly. Rola, the oldest, was a self-possessed young woman with a warm, round face. She was finishing her medical training, and it was a special treat for me tell her of her grandfather, Albert, the physician. Yara, the younger daughter, a dancer, had the lithe, dark beauty one imagines for Bizet's Carmen or Hugo's Esmeralda. The youngest child, Imad, was a tall young man and just beginning college. He was a real computer geek, and like so many his age around the world, he was fascinated by all things American. He insisted that Allen speak to him in English, a language in which both my nieces and my nephew were comfortable (along, of course, with Arabic and French).

After supper, Imad escorted us downstairs to our private bedroom, next to an attached bathroom. We slept in separate beds. The first few days in Lebanon, I managed to shower, but after that, showering became too cumbersome. Instead I sprayed myself with perfumed waters I purchased on the plane. Allen reassured me I did not smell. It is amazing how one can become accustomed to not showering daily.

The next morning, we awakened late. We headed upstairs. Halim and Mimo were there to greet us. We sat around the dining table as her Filipina live-in helper served us breakfast: fresh Lebanese bread like the bread I used to eat on our farm in Deir-el-Amar—thin, round, folded in half or quarters. My memories began to awaken. How was that possible? I had thought them dead and buried for decades. But, no, they were fighting their way to the surface.

Later, the four of us (Mimo and Halim, Allen and myself) got into Halim's van and headed for Notre Dame du Liban. Unfortunately, I could not make it to the top of that magnificent edifice. The climb is a steep, spiral ramp, at the top of which stands the statue of Notre Dame. There was no way a wheelchair could make it up. I had, fortunately, visited the site as a child, and while the others walked up the spiral, I simply prayed to Our Lady. The sunset and subsequent darkness gave us a spectacular view of the lights of the port of Jounieh far below.

That night, Halim drove north on the coastal highway. Rola was at work in the hospital, but she knew where we were heading, as did, apparently, the other family members. Halim finally stopped in front of a restaurant on the Mediterranean. We were in the ancient Phonecian city of Byblos. A huge, steep staircase stared at me as I sat in my wheelchair. No problem. Two young men working in the restaurant lifted up the wheelchair effortlessly, as though it were a feather, descended the steps, and placed me at the end of a long table that sat directly on the edge of the water. I could hear the Mediterranean caressing the rocks ever so gently below me.

We were not given menus, and no orders were taken. The feast simply began with the usual appetizers: *hummus, baba ghannouj, tabbouleh.* Then came the fresh fish, crispy and delicious. Mama Hana was with us, and she and I sat opposite each other, directly on the water's edge. At a certain point, Mimo addressed Allen, the only blue-eyed, pale-faced foreigner at the table, in French. She asked if he knew what dish the waiter had just placed in front of him. With a triumphant grin, Allen replied in Arabic: *akhtaboot* (octopus).

I could not help but listen to the Mediterranean serenading me. My emotions ran so deep that I have trouble describing them. There was a large hole in my psyche: my brother Tino's absence. I could only imagine how happy he would have been, surrounded by a family we thought we had lost forever.

I would have loved to drink some arak, but liquor was forbidden due to the daily drugs I had to ingest for my complex PTSD. But I smelled the arak, and that was enough to take me back decades. The quality of the food rivaled that in my memory. The conversations crossed linguistic barriers from Arabic through French, with a little English thrown in. How many hours did we sit by the water? However long it was, I knew it would never be enough. Yara got up from her chair at one point, came over to my side of the table, hugged me, and sat on the railing over the lapping sea. Her long black hair reached over her shoulders to the middle of her back, and if I had not known better, I would have taken her for a beautiful mermaid who had jumped out of the water to welcome my soul back to its native shore.

Time had no meaning. What I do remember is that the end of dinner was announced when Halim ordered *narghilas*. Everyone partook of them. I remember how shocked I was by seeing Mama Hana puffing away at her *narghila*, directly across from me.

I did not want the evening to end, but we soon found ourselves heading back to Mimo's house. I had only drunk sparkling water, but I was intoxicated. I actually had a family. For decades, my family was that of Allen. His mother treated me like a daughter and a friend. I loved and esteemed her. I never imagined that I would find my Lebanese family after all the decades of separation. They were mythical creatures to me, individuals I had hoped I would see again before I died but was never certain I would. Yet, there we were on the shore of my beloved Mediterranean.

When I arrived upstairs on the first day in Mimo's house, I had spotted an enormous framed picture of Christ on the Mount of Olives, in which Jesus is sitting and looking into the distance. There was nothing aesthetically remarkable about the painting, yet I could not take my eyes off it. It pulled me in like a magnet, and I simply gazed and gazed at it.

At a certain point, I asked Mimo if she would mind my seeing the picture up close. Of course not, she replied, taking it off the wall and bringing it to the dining room table, where I could drown myself in it. She explained that the picture had been recovered from what had been my father and Hana's bedroom. That must have been why it spoke to my unconscious memory.

I gazed at the picture and its frame, turning it over. Only then did I spot a large calling card attached to a corner of the frame. I called Mimo over and pointed the card out to her. Had she seen it before? She did not say, but she pulled out the card, and there in an elegant French cursive were words addressed to Papa (Dr. Albert Malti) from the Mother Superior at les Soeurs de St. Joseph, thanking my father for his gift. Mimo shrugged her shoulders and added that she had no idea what the card was about.

I explained to her that while I was a boarder with the Soeurs de St. Joseph, Papa had had a replica of the grotto at Lourdes built in the large school courtyard. Mimo said nothing, but I could see the shock on her face. She knew I wanted to go to my village of Deir el-Amar, and she promised we would stop at the convent where I went to school.

In truth, Mimo was not at all fond of our father. She was too young when he died to have any real memory of him, but that did not stop her from being angry at her missing parent. She would repeat over and over that she could never understand how the father of a family could leave his wife and children with nothing. Mama Hana explained it. My father had apparently written a will before he had gone to France to do his medical studies, leaving his worldly goods to his brother Michel. That would have been before he married Mama Odette as well as before he annulled that marriage and then married Mama Hana, whom he left with a two-or-three-year-old girl, Mimo. That original will was in the hands of Papa's friend, a physician from the prominent Khalidi family in Beirut, so Mama Hana went to meet Khalidi with my Uncle Michel after my father's demise. She argued strongly in favor of herself and her child as well as in favor of me and Constantine, but to no avail. The will had been written and had never been updated, and we were all left with nothing. Michel sold the enormous house, the farm, the land, the cisterns of water, the multiple fruit orchards (figs, apricots, oranges, and others)—everything that my father possessed—and kept the money. Mama Hana went back to her village of Ayn Zhalta and eventually married a member of the prominent Saad family.

During my visit to Lebanon, Mama Hana would tell me repeatedly how she could not understand my father's actions. Frankly, neither can I. It did suggest to me, however, how my Uncle Michel's purchase of a fancy home in Miami might have been possible. Needless to say, neither Costy nor I ever saw a penny from our father's estate.

To regret the past is to live in it. There are only so many tears one can shed over what did or did not take place. Mimo, true to her word, took us to Deir el-Amar. Alas, I had forgotten about the streets. They were narrow, made of large stones patched one next to the other, with a wide gutter in the middle of each street to direct flowing water, and impossible for a wheelchair to navigate. Halim drove to a spot below my street, where an older woman came out to greet me. She remembered me as a child. The visit was painful for both Mimo and me, but for me it was important because it reassured me that I had not imagined my past.

We headed for Les Soeurs de St. Joseph. The replica of Lourdes was in a sorry state. The blue belt on the Virgin Mary showed serious signs of age, and little Bernadette, kneeling before the Virgin, bore marks all over her body. But I could still read the text, "gift of Dr. A. G. Malti." My childhood was not a fantasy. I would have loved to spend more time, to visit my old school, but for Mimo, Deir al-Amar was a site of painful memories. She and Hana spent months in the house without enough money to get by, fighting with Aunt Najla. Hana even claimed that Najla sold goods without telling them and sent the money to Michel in America. After only a few hours, we left my childhood village, the site of so much family pain.

***

We took the road that led out of Deir al-Amar to visit my childhood friend, Marie Eid. Marie Eid was the last witness of my life in Deir el-Amar. Mimo had done some research and discovered that Marie had married her childhood sweetheart, Mousa, a stone mason. Mousa had built a castle made of stone with his own hands. He had lovingly carved each piece with different designs. Qasr Mousa, it was called (Mousa's castle). Halim, with his incredible patience, drove us to Qasr Mousa, which was a short distance down the road from Deir al-Amar. We were met by a herd of tour buses, lined up one next to another. There were so many tourists that I almost gave up hope of seeing my childhood friend.

But I did not give up. I grabbed someone who looked like he belonged at the site (a ticket taker, perhaps) and asked him if Madame Marie was there. Yes, he assured me, in Arabic. So I asked him to please go into the castle and tell Marie that her childhood friend Fedwa was there and wanted to see her. We waited and waited. I could see the impatience not only in Halim but in Mimo as well. Finally, out came my friend, Marie, dressed in black. I dared not ask whom she was mourning. I screamed out her name, and she screamed out mine as we were both fighting through the crowds. Before I knew it, we were hugging and kissing each other. I introduced Allen, Mimo, and Halim, but Marie and I were already back in time, in our childhood days.

"We were born on the same day," Marie announced to Mimo, who by now looked quite impatient. I did not remember that fact. No matter. We were inseparable as children. We were inseparable at school. The cruel thief who separated us was the one who stole my father's life. I kept telling Marie how much I missed her, and she said the same to me. Fortune was good to me that day. I wondered if she remembered how we checked our breasts while sitting on the bench at the entry to our house, next to my father's clinic. I did not ask. I told Marie that I hoped we would see each other again. She responded that if we did not see each other in this life, we would be reunited in Heaven.

That evening, we went to dinner at Yammina, a restaurant in Ayn Zhalta, the village where Mimo spent most of her childhood. At the restaurant, an enormous table awaited us. The owner knew Halim, Mimo, and the entire extended family. Relatives, more relatives, and still more relatives arrived. Every seat was filled, and the owner had to squeeze in more. I was overwhelmed by the number of family members I had no idea existed. Each woman was more beautiful than the last. The men were handsome and full of life. How was it possible that all these decades in America—when Costy and I were beaten and when I felt like a complete freak—could have passed without an inkling that we had a real family that existed independent of us in Lebanon? Marriages had taken place, children had been born and grown up, and babies were still on the way. Even more amazing to me was that everyone seated at the table seemed happy. Conversations that had started at one end of the table seemed to magically fly to other parts of the table, where the chatter continued.

So many dishes had arrived that the table itself virtually disappeared. All the appetizers and main dishes that had lived in my memory for decades greeted me like old friends. There was *kibbee nayee* (raw *kibbee*) with fresh onions, *baba ghannouj* (grilled eggplant with tahini sauce), baked *kibbee* in enormous pans cut into those lovely diamonds that dish always features, *kofta*, lamb shish kabob, fresh yogurt with fresh mint leaves, and rice with vermicelli.

Allen was sitting next to Mimo, who by then had noticed his predilection for unusual food. By contrast, as I have grown older, my tastes have altered to the point that I am almost a vegetarian. (I did not partake of either the raw *kibee* or the *kofta*, and certainly not the Lebanese sausage, a distant descendant of the sausage of my childhood encounter.) Mimo ordered a plate of tiny birds with all their body parts attached, which had been fried whole. As an American, Allen is not used to eating something whose head looks back at you, so he hid their faces by wrapping them in thin Arabic bread. He reported that they were crunchy and delicious, tasting of a kind of barbecue sauce perfumed with pomegranate.

As soon as Mimo realized that Allen was a voracious gourmet who was willing to try almost anything, she ordered a local specialty: morsels of raw sheep's liver, served with equal-sized pieces of raw sheep's fat. Mimo explained that this delicacy should be consumed with its "four spices": cumin, coriander, black pepper, and cayenne pepper. For Allen, this was more than a challenge because he normally does not eat liver, let alone raw liver. He wrapped the liver and fat, with their four spices, in bread. The result, he told me, was like a French paté or terrine. He asked me if I wanted a bite. "No, thank you," was my answer. I turned away and immersed myself in a conversation with my neighbors on the other side.

How many hours did we sit at Yammina? All I know is that we arrived in the late afternoon when it was still light outside and stayed as the sun ceded its place to the moon and day turned into night. After our feast, the staff at Yammina brought *narghilas*. The men partook, and the women partook. For the first time in my life, I noticed that each person was given a small mouthpiece to attach to the *narghila*, through which he or she would inhale the smoke. When they finished, they removed their piece and passed the *narghila* to the next guest, who would in turn attach his or her mouthpiece and puff away. I had noticed this taking place when we had dined on the seashore, but I had not paid it much mind. I did not remember this from my childhood, when I assumed that when the *narghila* was passed around, it was touched by multiple mouths. I did not partake of the *narghila*; I did not have to. Everything about the meal—the food, the sounds of laughter and clinking dinnerware, the sense of being part of a huge, vibrant, happy family—intoxicated me far beyond the power of mere tobacco smoke.

CHAPTER 36

Dreams of Flying

One evening, we were invited to Shadi and Rita's house for dinner. Shadi is Mimo's half-brother, the son of Mama Hana and her second husband. Mimo treats him as her brother, and so do I, as the other brother I did not even know I had. Rita, Shadi's wife, is a daughter of the Rahbany family. The Rahbany brothers, as they are known, are the biggest producers and composers of popular music in Lebanon and among the best known in the Arab world generally. Their most famous client is the Lebanese singer, Fairuz, also a worldwide celebrity. Shadi is the exclusive sound engineer for Fairuz in all her performances around the world. On Pope Benedict's trip to Lebanon in 2012, Shadi handled the audio, and he and his entire family, including Halim, Mimo, and their children, had front row seats at all the Papal functions.

I was completely seduced by the space in which Shadi and Rita lived in Beirut, a much more modern apartment than that of Mimo and Halim. With its clean lines, white walls, and beautiful furnishings, it could have passed for an Upper East Side apartment featured in the Design or Style sections of *The New York Times*. The dinner was served by a young woman who worked in Rita's home, and the food was exquisite: roast chicken on a bed of rice with pistachios and those golden raisins the French call "*raisins de Smyrne*" and which, in this case, really might have come from that Turkish city. In place of arak, Shadi served a selection of the finest wines from the western slope of Lebanon's Bekaa Valley.

Mama Hana was there, as were Rita's mother, Shadi, and Rita's two adorable boys. The older one was just learning to speak and called me Febwa (with a B) as he sat in my lap. His parents tried to correct him, but for me, the mispronunciation carried an innocent childlike affection. As he is getting older he says my name correctly, but I will always miss that adorable "Febwa."

The evening we spent at their home went by much too quickly. Mimo insisted that they show us a video of their wedding. It was not your normal wedding. It was a special occasion replete with an orchestra and a dance troupe in a performance in which every move had been choreographed. Rita was stunning, as was Shadi. I sat absolutely transfixed by the music, the gallantry, the complex ceremony. This event reminded me more of a royal wedding than a traditional marriage. Shadi explained that the musicians and dancers were Fairuz's professional company. Except that it was in color, the video at times resembled a 1930s Hollywood musical.

The evening at Shadi's brought home to me the magnitude of Mama Hana's achievement. Still a girl when she married my father, she was left a few short years later with no money and a young child to support. Hana somehow managed to get a job teaching while she completed her higher education. She supported her family, returned to her village of Ayn Zhalta, and married Mr. Saad, with whom she had a son. Mimo grew up to be a leading music teacher who travels around Lebanon, supervising other music instructors in the Lebanese school system. She married Halim, another high-school teacher, but when the Lebanese Civil War disrupted his career, Halim became a businessman and now runs his own prosperous insurance brokerage firm. Their three children, Hana's grandchildren, are as happy, healthy, and poised a group of young people as I have ever met.

***

The next day, we headed for downtown Beirut. We had Skyped Tino the night before to make sure that I had all the necessary information for the gold chain that I promised to purchase for him and on which he could hang his heavy cross. Everyone had a chance to speak to him: Rola, Yara, Imad, Halim, Mimo, Allen, and me. It was a strange sensation—all of us on Mimo's terrace being beamed into Tino's room. Since Allen and I are far less advanced in all things digital than either Costy or my Lebanese family, we had never Skyped anyone before. This, of course, was the two-way television that Najla and the womenfolk of the village had imagined before we left for America. I could see how neatly my brother kept his apartment, with Native American artifacts on the walls. (I am embarrassed to admit we had never visited him in Florida.) He looked excited to see all of us. I felt doubly guilty that he could not be with us.

On the way to Beirut, I asked Mimo if she minded our visiting my old boarding school of Les Soeurs de Besançon. We decided to go to the gold *souk* first. When we arrived there, I was astounded when we walked around it. It seemed so small compared to gold markets in other Middle Eastern cities. Had women in Lebanon stopped wearing so much gold on their arms? As I thought about it, I realized that

Mimo wore no gold at all, and neither did Mama Hana. The errand did not last long; we purchased a gold chain for Tino and two gold bangles for me.

I marveled at Halim's patience. He was willing to drive around and around the Beirut streets, with all the traffic. He had a rough idea where the convent of the Soeurs de Besançon was located. The problem was the many one-way streets. At last we arrived, only to find the gate locked. There was no way for us to enter the grounds. I put my head against the metal rails and looked around, trying to feast my eyes on as much of the site as I could. The majestic stairs leading to the building greeted me, as did the palm trees resting in a small area of the garden. It all looked so much smaller than I remembered. I told myself that my memory was playing tricks on me.

Suddenly, a dark sedan drove up next to Halim's SUV, and a nun wearing a habit came out from behind the wheel. She stared at us strangely, and immediately Mimo began to explain who we were and that I had been a boarder at the school when I was young. The nun took out her keys and unlocked the gate, inviting us into the garden. It was obvious that sitting in a wheelchair, as I was, I could not climb the majestic stairs.

The nun began asking me and Mimo questions. I told her my entire history with Les Soeurs de Besançon. She said she was ecstatic to have met someone like me. I asked her why the garden seemed so small to me and how I remembered that we girls used to run around that large open area and jump rope there. Unfortunately, she explained, commercial buildings had encroached on the area (something I had already noticed) after the school had been forced to sell off part of its property.

I could tell that Allen and Halim were both becoming impatient, but I was in another world, overwhelmed by memories and emotions. Suddenly, the nun asked me how long I would be in Lebanon. Unfortunately, I explained, a few days were all we had left of our one-week visit. She expressed her regret at my not having been there earlier that week, since she hosted a television program and would have loved to have me appear on it.

I find it difficult to describe how I felt on these all-too-brief visits. My desire to spend more time in my native country was overwhelming. I could have spoken to that nun for hours. I would have loved to know how she had garnered a spot on Lebanese television. I could have sat for hours and talked about how Papa always bought me a Tintin album from a store near the school and about my inability to jump over the rope in the enormous garden that had since disappeared. Alas, there was no way to revive the past, and Allen was giving me not-so-subtle signals that Halim was anxious to return home. I kissed the nun on both cheeks, something I would never have dared to do as a child, and I suspect she could see the emotion in my eyes. She made me promise to tell her the next time I was in Beirut so that I could appear on her show.

***

Someone decided that the next family excursion would be to the famous Jeita Grotto. I had never been there, but it is one of the most famous sites in Lebanon, and had been shortlisted for one of the Seven Wonders of the World. Halim drove us to the parking lot, where we boarded a tram (Halim and Allen hoisted me into the car). At the entrance to the cavern, I got back into my wheelchair, pushed by Imad (except for the few flights of stairs inside the cave, where two to three males lifted the chair over the obstacles). Imad led me through one of the most spectacular sites I have ever seen in my life. It was like being in an enormous cathedral with stalagmites and stalactites hanging from the ceiling above you, and once in a while blessing you with a drop of water. If one were to imagine a Heaven made of rock, this would be it. The colors of the stones varied and at every turn, and I would ask Imad to stop and just let me meditate for a moment. I have been in numerous houses of worship around the world, but there was a spirituality to this natural spot I had never encountered before in my life. I would have been ecstatic if I had had the opportunity to spend days, weeks—no, months—losing myself in that space.

We returned home, and that night Imad, who had watched me closely at the Grotto, asked me if I had ever seen the movie *Avatar*. No, I said. So he went out and purchased a disk (made illegally, of course, in Beirut), and the whole family gathered in the downstairs living room with its enormous screen. The first disk Imad bought was a dud. "No problem," he said. Before I knew it, he had returned with another copy of the film. This one worked. When I expressed my astonishment, he laughed and said this was completely normal in Beirut. You could buy anything, and if it didn't work, the merchant would simply give you another one.

It was as if Imad had been reading my mind while we were in Jeita. *Avatar* took me by the hand and continued the emotional journey I had experienced in the Grotto: the ethereal creatures flying through it and the handicapped American whose disability disappears as he moves about the jungle, flying free from tree to tree. I was emotionally spent. I wanted to watch the movie again and again. I wanted to lose myself in Jeita again and again, but I could do none of this in the real world.

***

The next morning, when we arrived upstairs, Mimo was there with a group of female teachers. She told Allen that he should join Halim, who was waiting to take him to his office. Meanwhile, Mimo and I would sit with the other women, drink coffee, eat pastry, and gossip. This was a weekly ritual, Mimo told me, a *subhiyya*, a morning get-together just for women—no men allowed. We sat around the dining room table and began gossiping. No subject was taboo—families, jobs, colleagues. When one cup of coffee was emptied, another reappeared from the kitchen. We sat at the table all morning and just talked. The conversations were not terribly deep, but I do not believe I ever worked in a university where the women professors in a department got together once a week to gossip. I realized how much sociability we lacked in the United States, and how I missed it.

***

Was it the next day? I am not sure. But I will never forget an experience in Lebanon that seemed another of those odd connections, those overlong strings desperately trying to tie my life together. We took a long car drive, over ranges of mountains, to the Mount Lebanon region in the north of the country, a landscape that I must surely have visited but cannot remember. We arrived at a mountaintop, a fairy-tale location floating over clouds below us. This is the sanctuary, I learn, of the Lebanese Maronite Saint Charbel (Mar Charbel in Syriac).

As a child, I had never heard of Mar Charbel. I encountered the name for the first time only two years before the Lebanon trip, in 2008, and not in Lebanon, but in Mexico City, in the Sonora market where I had gone to receive an exorcism—an attempt to drive the PTSD from my head. The market was filled with throngs of people milling around stands selling exotic spices and sacrificial animals such as black-skinned cocks with charcoal feathers. *La Santa Muerta* (Holy Death), cult of the drug traffickers, glared from painted skulls and draped skeletal figures.

After the exorcism, a book caught my eye. The cover was a shiny white and featured a picture of a religious figure. I felt drawn to this holy man. Eduardo, our guide and driver, told me it was Saint Charbel. Outside the market, a table sold little pious biographies of the saint in Spanish. Allen and I skimmed them to find some Mexican connection. There was none. Charbel lived and died in Lebanon. I bought the pamphlets but gave no further thought to this cultural transplant.

Two years later, I was stunned to find myself in Mar Charbel's shrine in the Lebanese mountains, along with Halim, Mimo, Allen, Imad, and Yara. The hermitage sits atop a mountain path, a challenge for my wheelchair because the car had been left in a distant parking lot. A multi-man team pushed me up the mountainside: husband, nephew, brother-in-law. The terrain was rocky, my team out of breath. Familiar feelings feasted on my brain—guilt at being a burden and shame over my physical state. My mouth engaged its refrain, "I'm sorry—I'm sorry—I'm sorry." My brother-in-law was breathing hard. I was praying silently that I had caused him no harm.

My sister walked behind us, barefoot on the rocky hillside, part of a vow she made to the Virgin Mary after a car accident had robbed her of some vertebrae, making her unable to stand or walk. Mimo had promised the Virgin, were she to cure her, that she would walk barefoot through all sanctuaries. I can see Mimo's face as she walks alone—calm, serene—in silent prayer.

The climb ended in a large square, where a gentleman greeted us. The painful trek, he revealed, was not necessary. If the guard had been at his post, he would have signaled us to proceed in the van. The descent, he assured us, would be much easier. No matter—we were in the presence of the Holy. A small sanctuary welcomed us. We lit candles. Now I know that these are the monks Costy and I visited in the mountains as children.

I sat in the wheelchair, Allen beside me, his hand in mine. I prayed, eyes closed, tears wetting my face. Did Mar Charbel hear my prayers? As if in answer, the Saint interceded. My eyes still closed, I felt the world disappearing and was suddenly aware that my seated body was floating above the wheelchair, free of this cumbersome machine. I was free. My arms rose along with my body, and I was free. I felt unattached to the world around me. I was afloat in one of those light blue clouds that surrounded Mar Charbel's hermitage.

We remained in the little chapel. I never wanted to leave. But the family had gone. Allen looked at my face. I wondered whether I dared share this. Allen assured me that I had experienced something neither of us could define. I never told Halim or Mimo. I was not looking for Mar Charbel. It was as if he found me.

CHAPTER 37

Tamriyya

Our last night in Beirut was magical. Mimo had invited the entire family to her home, including Halim's family, along with friends and other guests. For the trip, I had packed my traditional black outfits that I wore daily in the United States. It did not occur to me that people in the Middle East would interpret this clothing as a sign of mourning. I had to reassure them over and over again that no, women in America wore black all the time. On the last night, I decided to wear a light blue Harley-Davidson t-shirt replete with rhinestones over my black silk shirt.

Allen and I went upstairs to the living room, where our goodbye party was in full swing. The place was packed with family members, distant relatives, and close friends. Then a couple walked in and introduced themselves. The woman offered me a scarf as a gift, and her husband took out a book about a Lebanese political party, which was the party of the Jumblatt family (the left-of-center Progressive Socialist Party). He opened to the last page and showed me Papa's name along with the other founders of the organization. This affiliation surprised me. Though Papa and I had never talked politics, I had assumed, given his devout Catholicism and French associations, that he would be allied with right-of-center Christian parties, not a leftist Druze-based movement. A *Who's Who in Lebanon* listed him as without party, but there it was. He was a more complicated man than I had guessed. I asked for a copy of the book, but the man said this was his only copy. So be it: I had grown accustomed to losing family and any goods relating to them.

As the crowd was building, there was barely any space for new guests, but everyone somehow managed to squeeze in. Suddenly, I spotted Joe, Halim's brother, who is the personal bodyguard for the Belgian ambassador in Beirut. Joe was a big guy, but he managed to dance his way through the crowd, holding an enormous platter over his head. He spotted me, walked over to me, and gave me a big hug. Then he placed the platter in front of me at the table, and I was overcome. It was the childhood pastry that had haunted me all these years.

When I had described my quest to recover this childhood treat, Mimo had explained that the pastry was called *tamriyya* and was a specialty of Deir al-Amar, especially prepared for the feast day of Sayyidat el-Telle (Our Lady of the Mountain). We made inquiries during our trip to the village but were told that the old man who knew the recipe was near death. I had accepted that this would be another piece of forever-lost childhood.

I asked Joe how he managed to get the *tamriyya*. Joe put his index finger over his mouth, as though he were keeping a secret. He refused to tell me how and where he had found the *tamriyya*. He hugged me and told me that he had done this for me. He had chased all over Beirut to find someone who knew how to make this pastry and had ordered an entire platter for the party.

I did not think I could feel any more emotions than I had already in my native country, but Joe's incredible gift set my tears flowing. He insisted on giving me a *tamriyya* himself, which I accepted graciously. As soon as I bit into it, my entire childhood, all the memories I had buried over the years, erupted yet again into my consciousness—that combination of crispiness and a smooth, subtle sweetness. I think it was Mama Hana who explained that the secret to a proper *tamriyya* was flavoring the filling with water of citron, that ancient fruit of the Eastern Mediterranean.

This time, I could not control my reaction. There was no point in even trying. I hugged Joe again and thanked him over and over. He insisted I take a second *tamriyya*, which I did. Then I took a third and a fourth before stopping. I realized that I could not satiate myself with a past that had long disappeared, even if it meant eating a hundred *tamriyyas*.

Taste of *tamriyya*,
Altars of childhood,
Locked in memory,
Found and lost again.

CHAPTER 38

Refuge

I talk on the phone regularly with Mimo and Halim and follow the extended family on Facebook. Shadi, in particular, posts his travels and performances around the Mediterranean. For a few months after our visit (in 2010), Allen and I thought that some members of the family, perhaps Mimo and Hana, might visit Constantine in Florida. We soon came to understand, however, that Mimo and Halim were reluctant to leave Lebanon.

The 1982 Israeli invasion of Lebanon culminated in a fierce battle between Syrian and Israeli forces in Mimo and Halim's home village of Ayn Zhalta, forcing them to flee. They returned to find their home completely looted. Everything was gone—not just valuable property, but also personal goods and mementos like wedding pictures. When Halim talks about it, his sense of personal violation is palpable. Mimo and Halim rebuilt their lives (Halim replaced his career as teacher with that of successful businessman), but the scars remain. Every time there is a car bombing in Beirut, Halim draws his family together into a protective ring. Any suggestion that family members travel, or that we come to visit, is met with the same refrain: later, after the situation calms down in Lebanon. Allen and I understand how unlikely this is in the near future.

The idea of Constantine going to Lebanon, an idea Allen cherished for some time, also seems increasingly remote. It is not just that Constantine, unlike Allen, hates to travel. My brother's state of physical dependence keeps getting greater. Since around 2010, he has needed someone to help him transfer from the wheelchair to the bed and from the bed to the wheelchair. (He also cannot bathe himself.) Recently, in 2014, he got into a dispute with the worker who was supposed to help him to bed. She left in a huff, and Constantine spent six nights sleeping (or trying to sleep) in his wheelchair. This was so physically ruinous that he had to be hospitalized and spent three weeks in rehabilitation. Allen tells me that he has reluctantly given up his dream of a family reunion for Costy. We are now helping him out financially, as I used to help my mother, and Allen and I have visited him twice in Florida.

My handsome brother,
Like a movie star,
Sits not on a throne
But in a wheelchair.
Wheelchair is crowded;
Three men sit with him:
Charcot-Marie-Tooth.
Famed neurologists
A curious trio,
    Inspecting body,
Keeping detailed notes
On the nerves' progress.
Iron man shoulders
To be admired,
But alas the rest
Is as predicted:
    Costy's hands like claws
    That challenge eating,
    Grabbing at the food
    Shoveled into mouth.
        Body rituals
        In the lower zones
        Resemble Greek myths
        Inflicted by gods.
    A body in form
    Can tackle limits.
    A body askew
    Is seen as a curse.
Charcot-Marie-Tooth,
Papa's gift to us.
Musical trio
Squatters in our nerves.
Yet brother's body
Plays a different tune,
Not a symphony
But a hard rock band.

***

After the 2010 trip to Lebanon, Allen and I returned to our lives in Indiana, but we were not so much living as surviving. In my bedroom, I would run the television all day with crime shows—*Law and Order* and *CSI* in their various permutations. Allen did the same with the TV in the living room, but in his case it was all news, history, and cooking channels. We were just holding on until we had earned enough money to retire. The financial point of liberation came at the end of 2012.

During our last years in Indiana, I had at least gotten back into my pool, where I worked out several times a week with a physical therapist. Allen, who sometimes seems more concerned about my physical wellbeing than I am, was adamant that any place we lived would need an indoor pool. That would mean building a new house and selling our old one.

But where would we live? During our trips to Bennington for my MFA residencies, we often took a car from La Guardia airport to Vermont. When we went through Dutchess County in the Hudson Valley, Allen always noted its beauty, reminiscing about summers there as a child. Allen also liked the idea of living in Vermont (he loved Bennington), but I nixed this. Vermont was too cold and too far from New York City. To both of us, the Hudson Valley seemed just about right.

In August 2011, shortly after I graduated from Bennington, I heard about a poetry workshop being organized at the Omega Institute in Rhinebeck, New York. I wanted to go, and Allen said that this would be a perfect time to look at land in Dutchess County, where Omega was located. I researched locations on the Web, scoured census data, and chose Rhinebeck Township as the place to live. My main editorial contact at MacMillan for the *Encyclopedia of Sex and Gender* had bought a weekend house with her husband just across the river and was happy to pass us her real estate agent. In one day, before the poetry workshop began, we found our spot and made an offer on a wooded lot hidden away on a quiet country road.

Of course, we had been through this process before—hiring an architect, choosing a builder, and building a house—but doing it at a distance was an added complication. Allen made several trips, and I accompanied him on some of them to review plans with the architects, meet with builders, and at the later stages, choose finishes and paint colors. On one trip, Allen poured holy water and oil that I had brought back from Notre Dame du Liban into the foundation while I took pictures. I also liked the fact that our builder wore a medal for Saint Joseph, patron of carpenters.

On August 14, 2013, we moved into our almost-finished home (homeowners know that a house is never finished). Since neither of us had outgrown our architectural obsessions, the new house, like the old one, had high ceilings (for Allen) and no large windows (for Fedwa). There was one big difference. Our architect in Indiana, a great believer in natural light, felt that every room should have at least two, preferably three, exposures. The result was a design like a capital letter I (or a capital H with a longer middle). But its glorious spaces (we learned that in architecture, light creates space) made for long journeys. Allen used to joke that our bedroom and our studies were in different time zones. For me, going from the bedroom to the dining room became increasingly tiring (I was mostly living holed up in the master bedroom, anyway). The new architect proposed a flow plan that minimized walking distances (our bedroom is now steps from almost every other room), creating a far more compact design.

Moving out of our house in Bloomington meant facing up to my hoarding, especially since the new house was smaller than the old one. Painfully, I forced my closets to disgorge their disordered contents, emptied the boxes that hid under my bed and cluttered my floors, assembling everything into piles of clothing on the living room floor. With the help of one of my physical therapists (I could not face this alone), I sorted through my overabundant possessions. I abandoned my remaining fancy shoes, the clothes that were now too big, and whatever else I could bring myself to part with. The spring and early summer of 2013 saw Allen drive carload after carload of clothing and personal effects to Goodwill. We hired a young man with a pickup truck to take multiple loads to the Bloomington dump. We gave old and excess furniture to Saint Vincent de Paul.

Unlike our Indiana abode, the Rhinebeck house had no stack room, just a few built-in bookshelves. For the last several years, I have read electronic books almost exclusively. I find them easier on my weak hands and aging eyes. Allen also prefers that I read ebooks because I can buy as many as I want without creating any clutter. I gave my classical Arabic library to Catholic University in Washington and sold many of my other books to a used-book dealer in Philadelphia. Allen packed the boxes and drove them to the FedEx store in Bloomington.

In Rhinebeck, I mostly stay at home, reading, writing, and drawing on my iPad. (I published a chapbook of visual poetry.) The televisions remain off, except when we watch the Vatican masses for Easter and Christmas. We take all our meals together and have dinner every night in the dining room, where

Allen serves us magnificent meals culled from the bounty of the Hudson Valley. Sometimes life imitates art. A novel I was reading (I read so many novels on my iPad that I often forget both the authors and titles) took place in the Hudson Valley, and a character spoke of seeking out Macoon apples. I mentioned this to Allen and, as it was fall, he found a local source. Every day for lunch, during the season, we split one of these huge red apples. The crisp, white flesh offers a complex flavor, delicately balanced between tart and sweet.

Our new house is not marred by hoarding. My floors are clear. I can walk into my walk-in closets. I am in recovery. Are Charcot and his friends still with me? Of course. Am I still dancing with PTSD? Yes. But sleeping at night is now a pleasure and not a burden. The past, I have come to understand, is an essential part of the future, albeit a past that must be tamed.

About the Author

Raised in a Lebanese mountain village, **Fedwa Malti-Douglas** came to America at the age of 13. After a rich academic career, Professor Malti-Douglas turned her attention to other muses, publishing a novel (*Hisland*, SUNY Press) in 1998, and poetry (including a chapbook of visual poetry). Fedwa's honors include the 1997 Kuwait Prize in Arts and Letters, and the 2014 National Humanities Medal, presented in 2015 by President Barack Obama.

www.ingramcontent.com/pod-product-compliance
Lightning Source LLC
Chambersburg PA
CBHW080919100426
42812CB00007B/2322